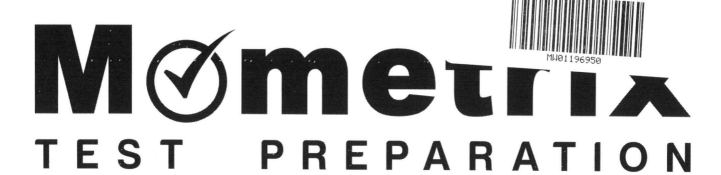

TEST PREPARATION

Dietetic Technician, Registered

Exam Secrets
Study Guide

Exam Review and DTR Practice Test
for the Dietetic Technician,
Registered Test

Written and edited by Mometrix Test Prep

Printed in the United States of America

This paper meets the requirements of ANSI/NISO Z39.48-1992 (Permanence of Paper).

Mometrix offers volume discount pricing to institutions. For more information or a price quote, please contact our sales department at sales@mometrix.com or 888-248-1219.

Mometrix Media LLC is not affiliated with or endorsed by any official testing organization. All organizational and test names are trademarks of their respective owners.

Paperback
ISBN 13: 978-1-5167-2317-1
ISBN 10: 1-5167-2317-1

DEAR FUTURE EXAM SUCCESS STORY

First of all, **THANK YOU** for purchasing Mometrix study materials!

Second, congratulations! You are one of the few determined test-takers who are committed to doing whatever it takes to excel on your exam. **You have come to the right place.** We developed these study materials with one goal in mind: to deliver you the information you need in a format that's concise and easy to use.

In addition to optimizing your guide for the content of the test, we've outlined our recommended steps for breaking down the preparation process into small, attainable goals so you can make sure you stay on track.

We've also analyzed the entire test-taking process, identifying the most common pitfalls and showing how you can overcome them and be ready for any curveball the test throws you.

Standardized testing is one of the biggest obstacles on your road to success, which only increases the importance of doing well in the high-pressure, high-stakes environment of test day. Your results on this test could have a significant impact on your future, and this guide provides the information and practical advice to help you achieve your full potential on test day.

Your success is our success

We would love to hear from you! If you would like to share the story of your exam success or if you have any questions or comments in regard to our products, please contact us at **800-673-8175** or **support@mometrix.com**.

Thanks again for your business and we wish you continued success!

Sincerely,
The Mometrix Test Preparation Team

> **Need more help? Check out our flashcards at:**
> **http://MometrixFlashcards.com/RD**

TABLE OF CONTENTS

Introduction

Thank you for purchasing this resource! You have made the choice to prepare yourself for a test that could have a huge impact on your future, and this guide is designed to help you be fully ready for test day. Obviously, it's important to have a solid understanding of the test material, but you also need to be prepared for the unique environment and stressors of the test, so that you can perform to the best of your abilities.

For this purpose, the first section that appears in this guide is the **Secret Keys**. We've devoted countless hours to meticulously researching what works and what doesn't, and we've boiled down our findings to the five most impactful steps you can take to improve your performance on the test. We start at the beginning with study planning and move through the preparation process, all the way to the testing strategies that will help you get the most out of what you know when you're finally sitting in front of the test.

We recommend that you start preparing for your test as far in advance as possible. However, if you've bought this guide as a last-minute study resource and only have a few days before your test, we recommend that you skip over the first two Secret Keys since they address a long-term study plan.

If you struggle with **test anxiety**, we strongly encourage you to check out our recommendations for how you can overcome it. Test anxiety is a formidable foe, but it can be beaten, and we want to make sure you have the tools you need to defeat it.

Secret Key #1 – Plan Big, Study Small

There's a lot riding on your performance. If you want to ace this test, you're going to need to keep your skills sharp and the material fresh in your mind. You need a plan that lets you review everything you need to know while still fitting in your schedule. We'll break this strategy down into three categories.

Information Organization

Start with the information you already have: the official test outline. From this, you can make a complete list of all the concepts you need to cover before the test. Organize these concepts into groups that can be studied together, and create a list of any related vocabulary you need to learn so you can brush up on any difficult terms. You'll want to keep this vocabulary list handy once you actually start studying since you may need to add to it along the way.

Time Management

Once you have your set of study concepts, decide how to spread them out over the time you have left before the test. Break your study plan into small, clear goals so you have a manageable task for each day and know exactly what you're doing. Then just focus on one small step at a time. When you manage your time this way, you don't need to spend hours at a time studying. Studying a small block of content for a short period each day helps you retain information better and avoid stressing over how much you have left to do. You can relax knowing that you have a plan to cover everything in time. In order for this strategy to be effective though, you have to start studying early and stick to your schedule. Avoid the exhaustion and futility that comes from last-minute cramming!

Study Environment

The environment you study in has a big impact on your learning. Studying in a coffee shop, while probably more enjoyable, is not likely to be as fruitful as studying in a quiet room. It's important to keep distractions to a minimum. You're only planning to study for a short block of time, so make the most of it. Don't pause to check your phone or get up to find a snack. It's also important to **avoid multitasking**. Research has consistently shown that multitasking will make your studying dramatically less effective. Your study area should also be comfortable and well-lit so you don't have the distraction of straining your eyes or sitting on an uncomfortable chair.

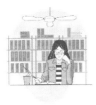 The time of day you study is also important. You want to be rested and alert. Don't wait until just before bedtime. Study when you'll be most likely to comprehend and remember. Even better, if you know what time of day your test will be, set that time aside for study. That way your brain will be used to working on that subject at that specific time and you'll have a better chance of recalling information.

Finally, it can be helpful to team up with others who are studying for the same test. Your actual studying should be done in as isolated an environment as possible, but the work of organizing the information and setting up the study plan can be divided up. In between study sessions, you can discuss with your teammates the concepts that you're all studying and quiz each other on the details. Just be sure that your teammates are as serious about the test as you are. If you find that your study time is being replaced with social time, you might need to find a new team.

2

Secret Key #2 – Make Your Studying Count

You're devoting a lot of time and effort to preparing for this test, so you want to be absolutely certain it will pay off. This means doing more than just reading the content and hoping you can remember it on test day. It's important to make every minute of study count. There are two main areas you can focus on to make your studying count.

Retention

It doesn't matter how much time you study if you can't remember the material. You need to make sure you are retaining the concepts. To check your retention of the information you're learning, try recalling it at later times with minimal prompting. Try carrying around flashcards and glance at one or two from time to time or ask a friend who's also studying for the test to quiz you.

To enhance your retention, look for ways to put the information into practice so that you can apply it rather than simply recalling it. If you're using the information in practical ways, it will be much easier to remember. Similarly, it helps to solidify a concept in your mind if you're not only reading it to yourself but also explaining it to someone else. Ask a friend to let you teach them about a concept you're a little shaky on (or speak aloud to an imaginary audience if necessary). As you try to summarize, define, give examples, and answer your friend's questions, you'll understand the concepts better and they will stay with you longer. Finally, step back for a big picture view and ask yourself how each piece of information fits with the whole subject. When you link the different concepts together and see them working together as a whole, it's easier to remember the individual components.

Finally, practice showing your work on any multi-step problems, even if you're just studying. Writing out each step you take to solve a problem will help solidify the process in your mind, and you'll be more likely to remember it during the test.

Modality

Modality simply refers to the means or method by which you study. Choosing a study modality that fits your own individual learning style is crucial. No two people learn best in exactly the same way, so it's important to know your strengths and use them to your advantage.

For example, if you learn best by visualization, focus on visualizing a concept in your mind and draw an image or a diagram. Try color-coding your notes, illustrating them, or creating symbols that will trigger your mind to recall a learned concept. If you learn best by hearing or discussing information, find a study partner who learns the same way or read aloud to yourself. Think about how to put the information in your own words. Imagine that you are giving a lecture on the topic and record yourself so you can listen to it later.

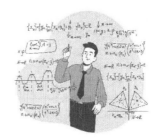

For any learning style, flashcards can be helpful. Organize the information so you can take advantage of spare moments to review. Underline key words or phrases. Use different colors for different categories. Mnemonic devices (such as creating a short list in which every item starts with the same letter) can also help with retention. Find what works best for you and use it to store the information in your mind most effectively and easily.

3

Secret Key #3 – Practice the Right Way

Your success on test day depends not only on how many hours you put into preparing, but also on whether you prepared the right way. It's good to check along the way to see if your studying is paying off. One of the most effective ways to do this is by taking practice tests to evaluate your progress. Practice tests are useful because they show exactly where you need to improve. Every time you take a practice test, pay special attention to these three groups of questions:

- The questions you got wrong
- The questions you had to guess on, even if you guessed right
- The questions you found difficult or slow to work through

This will show you exactly what your weak areas are, and where you need to devote more study time. Ask yourself why each of these questions gave you trouble. Was it because you didn't understand the material? Was it because you didn't remember the vocabulary? Do you need more repetitions on this type of question to build speed and confidence? Dig into those questions and figure out how you can strengthen your weak areas as you go back to review the material.

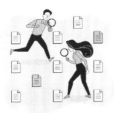 Additionally, many practice tests have a section explaining the answer choices. It can be tempting to read the explanation and think that you now have a good understanding of the concept. However, an explanation likely only covers part of the question's broader context. Even if the explanation makes perfect sense, **go back and investigate** every concept related to the question until you're positive you have a thorough understanding.

As you go along, keep in mind that the practice test is just that: practice. Memorizing these questions and answers will not be very helpful on the actual test because it is unlikely to have any of the same exact questions. If you only know the right answers to the sample questions, you won't be prepared for the real thing. **Study the concepts** until you understand them fully, and then you'll be able to answer any question that shows up on the test.

It's important to wait on the practice tests until you're ready. If you take a test on your first day of study, you may be overwhelmed by the amount of material covered and how much you need to learn. Work up to it gradually.

On test day, you'll need to be prepared for answering questions, managing your time, and using the test-taking strategies you've learned. It's a lot to balance, like a mental marathon that will have a big impact on your future. Like training for a marathon, you'll need to start slowly and work your way up. When test day arrives, you'll be ready.

Start with the strategies you've read in the first two Secret Keys—plan your course and study in the way that works best for you. If you have time, consider using multiple study resources to get different approaches to the same concepts. It can be helpful to see difficult concepts from more than one angle. Then find a good source for practice tests. Many times, the test website will suggest potential study resources or provide sample tests.

Practice Test Strategy

If you're able to find at least three practice tests, we recommend this strategy:

UNTIMED AND OPEN-BOOK PRACTICE

Take the first test with no time constraints and with your notes and study guide handy. Take your time and focus on applying the strategies you've learned.

TIMED AND OPEN-BOOK PRACTICE

Take the second practice test open-book as well, but set a timer and practice pacing yourself to finish in time.

TIMED AND CLOSED-BOOK PRACTICE

Take any other practice tests as if it were test day. Set a timer and put away your study materials. Sit at a table or desk in a quiet room, imagine yourself at the testing center, and answer questions as quickly and accurately as possible.

Keep repeating timed and closed-book tests on a regular basis until you run out of practice tests or it's time for the actual test. Your mind will be ready for the schedule and stress of test day, and you'll be able to focus on recalling the material you've learned.

Secret Key #4 – Pace Yourself

Once you're fully prepared for the material on the test, your biggest challenge on test day will be managing your time. Just knowing that the clock is ticking can make you panic even if you have plenty of time left. Work on pacing yourself so you can build confidence against the time constraints of the exam. Pacing is a difficult skill to master, especially in a high-pressure environment, so **practice is vital**.

Set time expectations for your pace based on how much time is available. For example, if a section has 60 questions and the time limit is 30 minutes, you know you have to average 30 seconds or less per question in order to answer them all. Although 30 seconds is the hard limit, set 25 seconds per question as your goal, so you reserve extra time to spend on harder questions. When you budget extra time for the harder questions, you no longer have any reason to stress when those questions take longer to answer.

Don't let this time expectation distract you from working through the test at a calm, steady pace, but keep it in mind so you don't spend too much time on any one question. Recognize that taking extra time on one question you don't understand may keep you from answering two that you do understand later in the test. If your time limit for a question is up and you're still not sure of the answer, mark it and move on, and come back to it later if the time and the test format allow. If the testing format doesn't allow you to return to earlier questions, just make an educated guess; then put it out of your mind and move on.

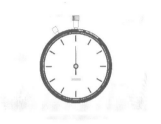

On the easier questions, be careful not to rush. It may seem wise to hurry through them so you have more time for the challenging ones, but it's not worth missing one if you know the concept and just didn't take the time to read the question fully. Work efficiently but make sure you understand the question and have looked at all of the answer choices, since more than one may seem right at first.

Even if you're paying attention to the time, you may find yourself a little behind at some point. You should speed up to get back on track, but do so wisely. Don't panic; just take a few seconds less on each question until you're caught up. Don't guess without thinking, but do look through the answer choices and eliminate any you know are wrong. If you can get down to two choices, it is often worthwhile to guess from those. Once you've chosen an answer, move on and don't dwell on any that you skipped or had to hurry through. If a question was taking too long, chances are it was one of the harder ones, so you weren't as likely to get it right anyway.

On the other hand, if you find yourself getting ahead of schedule, it may be beneficial to slow down a little. The more quickly you work, the more likely you are to make a careless mistake that will affect your score. You've budgeted time for each question, so don't be afraid to spend that time. Practice an efficient but careful pace to get the most out of the time you have.

Secret Key #5 – Have a Plan for Guessing

When you're taking the test, you may find yourself stuck on a question. Some of the answer choices seem better than others, but you don't see the one answer choice that is obviously correct. What do you do?

The scenario described above is very common, yet most test takers have not effectively prepared for it. Developing and practicing a plan for guessing may be one of the single most effective uses of your time as you get ready for the exam.

In developing your plan for guessing, there are three questions to address:

- When should you start the guessing process?
- How should you narrow down the choices?
- Which answer should you choose?

When to Start the Guessing Process

Unless your plan for guessing is to select C every time (which, despite its merits, is not what we recommend), you need to leave yourself enough time to apply your answer elimination strategies. Since you have a limited amount of time for each question, that means that if you're going to give yourself the best shot at guessing correctly, you have to decide quickly whether or not you will guess.

Of course, the best-case scenario is that you don't have to guess at all, so first, see if you can answer the question based on your knowledge of the subject and basic reasoning skills. Focus on the key words in the question and try to jog your memory of related topics. Give yourself a chance to bring the knowledge to mind, but once you realize that you don't have (or you can't access) the knowledge you need to answer the question, it's time to start the guessing process.

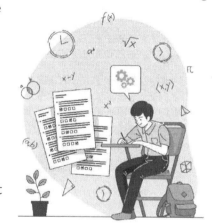

It's almost always better to start the guessing process too early than too late. It only takes a few seconds to remember something and answer the question from knowledge. Carefully eliminating wrong answer choices takes longer. Plus, going through the process of eliminating answer choices can actually help jog your memory.

Summary: Start the guessing process as soon as you decide that you can't answer the question based on your knowledge.

7

How to Narrow Down the Choices

The next chapter in this book (**Test-Taking Strategies**) includes a wide range of strategies for how to approach questions and how to look for answer choices to eliminate. You will definitely want to read those carefully, practice them, and figure out which ones work best for you. Here though, we're going to address a mindset rather than a particular strategy.

Your odds of guessing an answer correctly depend on how many options you are choosing from.

Number of options left	5	4	3	2	1
Odds of guessing correctly	20%	25%	33%	50%	100%

You can see from this chart just how valuable it is to be able to eliminate incorrect answers and make an educated guess, but there are two things that many test takers do that cause them to miss out on the benefits of guessing:

- Accidentally eliminating the correct answer
- Selecting an answer based on an impression

We'll look at the first one here, and the second one in the next section.

To avoid accidentally eliminating the correct answer, we recommend a thought exercise called **the $5 challenge**. In this challenge, you only eliminate an answer choice from contention if you are willing to bet $5 on it being wrong. Why $5? Five dollars is a small but not insignificant amount of money. It's an amount you could afford to lose but wouldn't want to throw away. And while losing

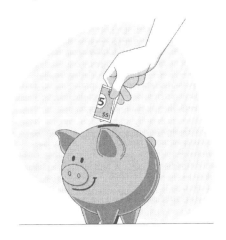

$5 once might not hurt too much, doing it twenty times will set you back $100. In the same way, each small decision you make—eliminating a choice here, guessing on a question there—won't by itself impact your score very much, but when you put them all together, they can make a big difference. By holding each answer choice elimination decision to a higher standard, you can reduce the risk of accidentally eliminating the correct answer.

The $5 challenge can also be applied in a positive sense: If you are willing to bet $5 that an answer choice *is* correct, go ahead and mark it as correct.

Summary: Only eliminate an answer choice if you are willing to bet $5 that it is wrong.

8

Which Answer to Choose

You're taking the test. You've run into a hard question and decided you'll have to guess. You've eliminated all the answer choices you're willing to bet $5 on. Now you have to pick an answer. Why do we even need to talk about this? Why can't you just pick whichever one you feel like when the time comes?

The answer to these questions is that if you don't come into the test with a plan, you'll rely on your impression to select an answer choice, and if you do that, you risk falling into a trap. The test writers know that everyone who takes their test will be guessing on some of the questions, so they intentionally write wrong answer choices to seem plausible. You still have to pick an answer though, and if the wrong answer choices are designed to look right, how can you ever be sure that you're not falling for their trap? The best solution we've found to this dilemma is to take the decision out of your hands entirely. Here is the process we recommend:

Once you've eliminated any choices that you are confident (willing to bet $5) are wrong, select the first remaining choice as your answer.

Whether you choose to select the first remaining choice, the second, or the last, the important thing is that you use some preselected standard. Using this approach guarantees that you will not be enticed into selecting an answer choice that looks right, because you are not basing your decision on how the answer choices look.

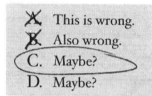

This is not meant to make you question your knowledge. Instead, it is to help you recognize the difference between your knowledge and your impressions. There's a huge difference between thinking an answer is right because of what you know, and thinking an answer is right because it looks or sounds like it should be right.

Summary: To ensure that your selection is appropriately random, make a predetermined selection from among all answer choices you have not eliminated.

Test-Taking Strategies

This section contains a list of test-taking strategies that you may find helpful as you work through the test. By taking what you know and applying logical thought, you can maximize your chances of answering any question correctly!

It is very important to realize that every question is different and every person is different: no single strategy will work on every question, and no single strategy will work for every person. That's why we've included all of them here, so you can try them out and determine which ones work best for different types of questions and which ones work best for you.

Question Strategies

⊘ READ CAREFULLY

Read the question and the answer choices carefully. Don't miss the question because you misread the terms. You have plenty of time to read each question thoroughly and make sure you understand what is being asked. Yet a happy medium must be attained, so don't waste too much time. You must read carefully and efficiently.

⊘ CONTEXTUAL CLUES

Look for contextual clues. If the question includes a word you are not familiar with, look at the immediate context for some indication of what the word might mean. Contextual clues can often give you all the information you need to decipher the meaning of an unfamiliar word. Even if you can't determine the meaning, you may be able to narrow down the possibilities enough to make a solid guess at the answer to the question.

⊘ PREFIXES

If you're having trouble with a word in the question or answer choices, try dissecting it. Take advantage of every clue that the word might include. Prefixes and suffixes can be a huge help. Usually, they allow you to determine a basic meaning. *Pre-* means before, *post-* means after, *pro-* is positive, *de-* is negative. From prefixes and suffixes, you can get an idea of the general meaning of the word and try to put it into context.

⊘ HEDGE WORDS

Watch out for critical hedge words, such as *likely, may, can, sometimes, often, almost, mostly, usually, generally, rarely,* and *sometimes.* Question writers insert these hedge phrases to cover every possibility. Often an answer choice will be wrong simply because it leaves no room for exception. Be on guard for answer choices that have definitive words such as *exactly* and *always.*

⊘ SWITCHBACK WORDS

Stay alert for *switchbacks.* These are the words and phrases frequently used to alert you to shifts in thought. The most common switchback words are *but, although,* and *however.* Others include *nevertheless, on the other hand, even though, while, in spite of, despite,* and *regardless of.* Switchback words are important to catch because they can change the direction of the question or an answer choice.

10

⊘ Face Value

When in doubt, use common sense. Accept the situation in the problem at face value. Don't read too much into it. These problems will not require you to make wild assumptions. If you have to go beyond creativity and warp time or space in order to have an answer choice fit the question, then you should move on and consider the other answer choices. These are normal problems rooted in reality. The applicable relationship or explanation may not be readily apparent, but it is there for you to figure out. Use your common sense to interpret anything that isn't clear.

Answer Choice Strategies

⊘ Answer Selection

The most thorough way to pick an answer choice is to identify and eliminate wrong answers until only one is left, then confirm it is the correct answer. Sometimes an answer choice may immediately seem right, but be careful. The test writers will usually put more than one reasonable answer choice on each question, so take a second to read all of them and make sure that the other choices are not equally obvious. As long as you have time left, it is better to read every answer choice than to pick the first one that looks right without checking the others.

⊘ Answer Choice Families

An answer choice family consists of two (in rare cases, three) answer choices that are very similar in construction and cannot all be true at the same time. If you see two answer choices that are direct opposites or parallels, one of them is usually the correct answer. For instance, if one answer choice says that quantity x increases and another either says that quantity x decreases (opposite) or says that quantity y increases (parallel), then those answer choices would fall into the same family. An answer choice that doesn't match the construction of the answer choice family is more likely to be incorrect. Most questions will not have answer choice families, but when they do appear, you should be prepared to recognize them.

⊘ Eliminate Answers

Eliminate answer choices as soon as you realize they are wrong, but make sure you consider all possibilities. If you are eliminating answer choices and realize that the last one you are left with is also wrong, don't panic. Start over and consider each choice again. There may be something you missed the first time that you will realize on the second pass.

⊘ Avoid Fact Traps

Don't be distracted by an answer choice that is factually true but doesn't answer the question. You are looking for the choice that answers the question. Stay focused on what the question is asking for so you don't accidentally pick an answer that is true but incorrect. Always go back to the question and make sure the answer choice you've selected actually answers the question and is not merely a true statement.

⊘ Extreme Statements

In general, you should avoid answers that put forth extreme actions as standard practice or proclaim controversial ideas as established fact. An answer choice that states the "process should be used in certain situations, if..." is much more likely to be correct than one that states the "process should be discontinued completely." The first is a calm rational statement and doesn't even make a definitive, uncompromising stance, using a hedge word *if* to provide wiggle room, whereas the second choice is far more extreme.

⊘ Benchmark

As you read through the answer choices and you come across one that seems to answer the question well, mentally select that answer choice. This is not your final answer, but it's the one that will help you evaluate the other answer choices. The one that you selected is your benchmark or standard for judging each of the other answer choices. Every other answer choice must be compared to your benchmark. That choice is correct until proven otherwise by another answer choice beating it. If you find a better answer, then that one becomes your new benchmark. Once you've decided that no other choice answers the question as well as your benchmark, you have your final answer.

⊘ Predict the Answer

Before you even start looking at the answer choices, it is often best to try to predict the answer. When you come up with the answer on your own, it is easier to avoid distractions and traps because you will know exactly what to look for. The right answer choice is unlikely to be word-for-word what you came up with, but it should be a close match. Even if you are confident that you have the right answer, you should still take the time to read each option before moving on.

General Strategies

⊘ Tough Questions

If you are stumped on a problem or it appears too hard or too difficult, don't waste time. Move on! Remember though, if you can quickly check for obviously incorrect answer choices, your chances of guessing correctly are greatly improved. Before you completely give up, at least try to knock out a couple of possible answers. Eliminate what you can and then guess at the remaining answer choices before moving on.

⊘ Check Your Work

Since you will probably not know every term listed and the answer to every question, it is important that you get credit for the ones that you do know. Don't miss any questions through careless mistakes. If at all possible, try to take a second to look back over your answer selection and make sure you've selected the correct answer choice and haven't made a costly careless mistake (such as marking an answer choice that you didn't mean to mark). This quick double check should more than pay for itself in caught mistakes for the time it costs.

⊘ Pace Yourself

It's easy to be overwhelmed when you're looking at a page full of questions; your mind is confused and full of random thoughts, and the clock is ticking down faster than you would like. Calm down and maintain the pace that you have set for yourself. Especially as you get down to the last few minutes of the test, don't let the small numbers on the clock make you panic. As long as you are on track by monitoring your pace, you are guaranteed to have time for each question.

⊘ Don't Rush

It is very easy to make errors when you are in a hurry. Maintaining a fast pace in answering questions is pointless if it makes you miss questions that you would have gotten right otherwise. Test writers like to include distracting information and wrong answers that seem right. Taking a little extra time to avoid careless mistakes can make all the difference in your test score. Find a pace that allows you to be confident in the answers that you select.

12

⌀ Keep Moving

Panicking will not help you pass the test, so do your best to stay calm and keep moving. Taking deep breaths and going through the answer elimination steps you practiced can help to break through a stress barrier and keep your pace.

Final Notes

The combination of a solid foundation of content knowledge and the confidence that comes from practicing your plan for applying that knowledge is the key to maximizing your performance on test day. As your foundation of content knowledge is built up and strengthened, you'll find that the strategies included in this chapter become more and more effective in helping you quickly sift through the distractions and traps of the test to isolate the correct answer.

Now that you're preparing to move forward into the test content chapters of this book, be sure to keep your goal in mind. As you read, think about how you will be able to apply this information on the test. If you've already seen sample questions for the test and you have an idea of the question format and style, try to come up with questions of your own that you can answer based on what you're reading. This will give you valuable practice applying your knowledge in the same ways you can expect to on test day.

Good luck and good studying!

Food and Nutrition Sciences

Principles of Food Preparation

PHYSICAL AND CHEMICAL PROPERTIES OF FOOD
FOOD ADDITIVES

Gras, Delaney clause and "no observable effect level"

GRAS means generally recognized as safe. This list was developed in 1958 to categorize food additives generally thought to be safe for consumption. U.S. congress felt that food manufacturers should not have to prove the safety of substances they already added to foods; instead this was deemed to be the responsibility of the FDA. Many chemicals on the GRAS list have not been rigorously tested because of the expense. Instead, these additives are generally thought to be safe because of their long history of safe use.

The *Delaney clause* was added to the 1958 Pure Food and Drug Act in the U.S. to ensure that food additives known to be carcinogenic to man or animals would not be used in food, regardless of the margin of safety.

The *"no observable effect level"* corresponds to the highest dose of a food additive that can be found to produce no adverse health effects in animals. This number is then used to establish a margin of safety for the use of the additive in human foodstuffs.

ANTIOXIDANTS, EMULSIFIERS, HUMECTANTS, AND PRESERVATIVES

Antioxidants such as BHA, BHT, and vitamin E function to maintain the freshness of foods by preventing fats from turning rancid and preventing discoloration.

Emulsifiers are used to improve the smoothness and uniformity of products like ice cream, pastries, and candies. They suspend and distribute fats or oils in liquids, and they can also function to stabilize fat and oil mixtures like mayonnaise to prevent the product from separating.

Humectants are often found in products like candy and shredded coconut, where they function to maintain moisture levels, freshness, and a desirable texture.

There are many types of preservatives, and their role includes preventing rancidity, inhibiting microbial growth, and preventing oxidation of foods. Nitrates and nitrites are commonly found in processed meats as a C. botulinum inhibitor. Other common preservatives include ascorbic acid, calcium propionate, sodium benzoate, and vitamin C.

EGGS
GRADING OF EGGS

The grading of eggs is governed by USDA standards, although it is not mandatory. The grades encompass both interior and exterior quality, and eggs may be assigned a grade of AA, A, or B. Grade AA eggs have the most superior quality, with firm yolks that stand up tall and thick whites that cling to the yolk area. Grade A eggs are most commonly found in the grocery store, and most consumers would not be able to discern a difference between A and AA eggs. Grade B eggs, although suitable for eating, are usually shipped to food manufacturers for use in recipes. The yolks appear flattened out and the whites are thin. Eggs are grouped for sale according to size, so that the weight of a dozen eggs meets the standard for that size. Six size equivalents offered for sale:

15

peewee (15 oz.), small (18 oz.), medium (21 oz.), large (24 oz.), extra-large (27 oz.), and jumbo (30 oz.). The standard size for recipe use is large.

NUTRITIVE VALUE

Eggs are considered a nutrient dense food, as they supply a large amount of nutrition in relation to the calories they contain. One large whole egg can provide over 10% of the daily recommended value of protein, including all of the amino acids essential to the body. The egg white, or albumen, is a high-quality, fat-free source of protein in the eggs. The white also contains about half of the vitamin and mineral content of the egg, making it a good source of niacin, riboflavin, potassium, and magnesium. The egg yolk contains all of the egg's fat, vitamin A, vitamin D, vitamin E, and zinc. The yolk is also the source of cholesterol in the egg, so egg yolks may be restricted for those on a low-cholesterol diet.

CHEESE

The making of cheese involves separating the curd from the whey in milk or cream, consolidating the curd, and usually ripening the final product. Coagulation disrupts the casein protein in the milk, causing a gel to form. Coagulation is facilitated by using enzymes, acid, or a combination of heat and acid. After the gel has been allowed to firm, the curds are cut into pieces, which begin to expel the liquid whey. Cooking helps to separate the whey from the curd, and also determines the final moisture content and pH level of the cheese. Most cheeses undergo a ripening process to achieve the desired body, texture, and flavor. Ripening agents cause the protein, fat, and lactose to break down. Common agents used include introduced molds, enzymes, rennet, and lipase. The ripening stage can take weeks, months, or even years, depending on the type of cheese.

DAIRY PROCESSING TECHNIQUES

Pasteurization is one of the most important steps in the production of milk products. The rationale for pasteurization is twofold: to destroy pathogens harmful to humans, and to extend shelf life by destroying bacteria that cause spoilage. The extent of pathogen destruction depends on the temperature and the length of exposure to the heat. UHT, or ultra-high temperature processing, takes this notion one step further by using temperatures in excess of boiling to render the product sterile. This results in a product with a shelf life of six months or longer, but the "cooked milk flavor" is a downside. Homogenization acts as a mechanical emulsifying process, suspending the fatty globules of whole milk in the water layer. Without this, the fat would rise to the top as cream. The fat globules are forced through an extruder to break them into smaller particles, and this smaller surface area allows the emulsion to stabilize.

MEAT AND POULTRY
FACTORS AFFECTING COLOR

Two pigments are primarily responsible for the color variations we see in meat and poultry: myoglobin and oxymyoglobin. Myoglobin produces the reddish-purple color seen in beef. When meat tissues are exposed to oxygen, oxymyoglobin is produced, which produces a bright red color. Therefore, meat products that are vacuum-sealed, and thus protected from oxygen exposure, will have a purplish-red appearance, while those meat products displayed in the butcher's case will have the bright red appearance characteristic of oxymyoglobin formation. Color is not a reliable indicator of freshness of meat or doneness in cooking. Using an instant read thermometer to ensure cooking temperatures have reached 160 degrees Fahrenheit throughout ensures the destruction of pathogens. Poultry can vary in appearance from white to yellowish-white to bluish white, depending on the feed used, age of the bird, and activity level of the bird. As with beef, color is not an indicator of doneness, and cooked temperatures of 165 degrees Fahrenheit should determine cooking times rather than relying on color.

16

INSPECTION AND GRADING PROCESS FOR BEEF

Inspection of meat for safety and wholesomeness is mandated by the federal government, while the grading process is a voluntary process beef manufacturers pay for. The Food Safety and Inspection Service (FSIS) is a branch of the USDA that inspects meat for safe processing, labeling, and packaging according to the Federal Meat Inspection Act. If meat is sold beyond the state in which it was produced, the state inspection system used must meet or exceed federal guidelines. The inspection process uses random sampling to uncover hidden dangers such as pathogens or chemical contamination, and meat that passes the testing process receives a round purple stamp. After receiving a passing mark for wholesomeness, a beef processing plant may wish to pay for the voluntary federal grading process. A high grade indicates the product meets standards for tenderness, juiciness, and flavor. The grades are then assigned as (in descending order of quality) prime, choice, or select.

DRY HEAT AND MOIST HEAT METHODS

Dry heat methods for preparing meat commonly include frying, broiling, grilling, and roasting. Cuts of meat close to the rib or loin have less connective tissue (collagen), and are the most suitable for these cooking methods. The USDA recommends that while hamburger products should be cooked to a temperature of 165 degrees F, whole muscle meats may be cooked to 145 degrees if rare beef is desired.

Moist heat cooking is a good way to utilize less expensive, tougher cuts of meat that come from the chuck or round. Weight bearing muscles contain more collagen, and older animals contain more collagen. Slow cooking methods of applying moist heat take advantage of the fact that collagen is soluble in water. Methods like stewing, simmering, braising, and steaming allow the collagen to gelatinize, tenderizing the meat.

SEAFOOD

The FDA is the governing body that oversees seafood products to ensure safety through its Hazard Analysis Critical Points Control Program. Rather than focusing on the finished seafood product to identify safety issues, this program seeks to identify and prevent problems that could cause illness in seafood. The U.S. Department of Commerce also runs a voluntary, fee-for-service program via the National Oceanic and Atmospheric Administration. This program goes beyond the basic safety assurances of the FDA program to further examine seafood for wholesomeness and quality. If the product meets the guidelines set forth by the U.S.D.C. for quality, the manufacturer is permitted to label the product as "grade A," indicating that the highest level of quality has been met. Unlike other food products inspected by the government for quality, there are no lesser grades for seafood.

BREADS
GLUTEN DEVELOPMENT

Many different flours are used in baking, but only wheat flour has enough of the protein gluten to contribute to structural changes in the final product. When gluten comes into contact with moisture the proteins adhere to water and form a web-like structure that exhibits elastic qualities. Mechanical manipulation such as kneading, beating, or stirring enhances gluten's ability to bind with water. After the gluten has reached the desired stage of development, the net-like structure functions to hold gas bubbles in the batter or dough, which makes gluten an important leavening agent. When the product encounters the heat of the oven, the moisture evaporates and the previously elastic gluten structure becomes rigid, yielding a baked good whose volume is stable. Different types of wheat flour have different gluten levels, and the choice of flour one uses depends of the desired texture of the final product. For example, more tender products such as cakes call for flour with lower gluten content.

RETROGRADATION IN STARCHES

Starch is composed of amylose and amylopectin, and those starches with a higher proportion of amylose are more prone to retrogradation. More waxy starches containing high amylopectin amounts, such as corn and rice, do not experience this problem. When starch is exposed to water and heat, the molecules swell and viscosity is increased; this is part of the gelatinization process. When the gel cools the starch may lose some of its ability to hold water, water is forced out of the gel, and syneresis or weeping of fluid can occur. The crystalline structure of the gel breaks down and the hydrogen bonds in the amylose recrystallize in a more orderly way. This results in a grainy product or a sauce that has a viscous layer surrounded by a puddle of water due to syneresis. Freezing exacerbates retrogradation and choosing waxy starch ingredients prevents the problem.

LEAVENING

Regardless of the method of leavening used in bakery products, the goal is the same: to produce carbon dioxide gas. Mechanical leavening takes place when air is incorporated into the batter or dough as a result of the mixing technique used. Egg whites are one of the primary mechanical leavening agents, as egg whites foam when beaten or whipped, trapping air bubbles in the batter. The proteins in the foam coagulate and stabilize in the presence of cooking temperatures. Steam can also contribute to volume in some products. Chemical leavening agents include baking soda and baking powder. Baking soda needs to come into contact with moisture and an acidic ingredient to be activated. Baking powder only needs moisture to release its leavening power. Yeast is considered a biological leavening product, as it is a live organism. The leavening occurs when the organism feeds off of the sugar or flour in the presence of moisture in the product and produces carbon dioxide and ethanol.

PIGMENTS

Changes that occur in plant pigments during the preparation of fruits and vegetables can increase or decrease the nutrient content and appeal of these foods.

Chlorophyll is the energy synthesizing molecule that gives plants their characteristic green color. The magnesium atom in chlorophyll is replaced with a hydrogen atom in the presence of acid, forming pheophytin and resulting in a drab olive color. Conversely, chlorophyll turns bright green in the presence of an alkaline solution.

Carotenoids are usually yellow, orange, or red, and include the well-known nutrient carotene, an important vitamin A precursor. Carotenes are insoluble in water, and they are also stable in an acid or alkaline solution, so cooking does little to reduce the bright color.

Flavonoids include the red and blue anthocyanins found in blueberries, which serve as an antioxidant in the diet. These water-soluble pigments turn bright red in the presence of acid, and take on a more bluish hue in the presence of alkaline solutions.

FRUIT RIPENING

The hormone ethylene is largely responsible for the ripening process in fruits. This gas passes through the air from one fruit to another and acts like an invisible signal to other fruits to begin to ripen and decay. The gas is produced in higher amounts by some fruits, such as apples, bananas, peaches, and pears, while other fruits, such as grapes, strawberries, and citrus fruits produce less of the gas. The gas is produced in higher amounts in reaction to certain environmental stresses, such as high temperatures and wounding. Growers have been able to use their knowledge of ethylene to their advantage, so that ethylene conditions in the warehouse may be perfectly controlled to determine the time at which peak ripeness occurs. Consumers can control the ripening effects of ethylene at home by storing most produce in the refrigerator and placing unripe produce on the counter to achieve peak flavor.

FOOD PREPARATION
COOKING TERMS

Al dente: A term used in reference to cooking pasta. It is translated from Italian to "to the tooth," and essentially means, slightly chewy.

Bake: The use of an oven for providing dry heat. Baking is most commonly used to prepare pastry goods, desserts, and casseroles.

Baste: Used to designate that moisture should be added to foods while they cook. Typically, basting is done using pan drippings that are poured over the top of the cooking item.

Beat: To beat an item means to mix it vigorously, often with a whisk or electric mixer.

Bard: Method of wrapping meat in fat before cooking.

Blackened: Cooking food in a Cajun style, where the food is generally heavily seasoned and then cooked over high heat until charred.

Blanching: Cooking method in which items are cooked using boiling water, by simmering or steaming a food or having the boiling water poured over the food.

Blend: Term for combining ingredients until they reach a smooth texture and consistency.

Boil: Cooking method in which a liquid is heated until it bubbles and breaks upon the surface of a liquid.

Braise: To cook food in a small amount of water or liquid while covered.

Broil: Method of cooking in which food is exposed to direct, dry heat. Broiling is often done in an oven or on a grill.

Brown: To cook food until the surface achieves a brown color. Browning may be done in some form of fat or oil and is often the first step in a longer cooking process.

Chop: Cutting term, in which food is cut using a knife, food processor, or other cutting instrument into small pieces.

Clarify: Method of skimming a food to remove fat from the surface and/or smaller pieces from remaining fat.

Cream: Mixing term in which butter or another fat is beaten until fluffy. Creaming may occur with or without an additional ingredient, such as sugar.

Cube: Cutting term in which food is cut into small, cubes.

Cut-in: Mixing a fat with dry ingredients until small crumb-like pieces are formed.

Deglaze: Making a sauce or gravy in which a small amount of liquid is added to a pan that meat was cooked in. As the liquid heats, the pan is scraped and the remaining food bits are combined with the liquid for flavorful sauce.

Dicing: A cutting term, which refers to cutting an item into small cubes, generally smaller than the particles that result from cubing an item.

Dissolve: To mix a solid into a liquid until a homogenous solution forms and no solid remains.

Dredge: To coat a food with flour, bread crumbs, or another food. Foods are often dredged before being fried.

Dust: Sprinkling seasoning or another dry ingredient on a food.

Fold: Gently blend ingredients to prevent over-beating or flattening items. Folding is usually done using a light rubber spatula to sweep down and across a mixture.

Fry: A cooking method in which food is cooked in highly heated oil or fat. Deep (fat) frying is when a food is submerged in the hot oil. When little oil is used, it is called sautéing or pan-frying.

Garnish: Dressing a plate, usually with an edible object, such as an herb, flower, chocolate or sauce. Garnish is both the act of dressing the plate as well as the term for the object dressing the plate.

Grate: A method of cutting food by rubbing it across a grater with the result being small shavings.

Grease: Preparing a pan for cooking or baking by coating it with a layer of fat. Greasing is generally done to prevent food from sticking to the pan.

Julienne: A method of cutting in which food is cut into thin strips that are approximately the size of matches.

Knead: Developing gluten in yeast breads. Kneading is done by folding and pressing down on dough until it results in a smooth texture.

Macerate: Soaking fruits or vegetables in a liquid.

Marinate: Soaking meat in liquid in order to flavor and/or tenderize it.

Mince: To chop food into very small, irregular pieces.

Pare: To peel the skin from a fruit or vegetable using a knife and/or a peeler.

Poach: A cooking method in which a food is cooked in simmering water or another liquid.

Preheat: The step in the cooking process in which the cook prepares the oven (or other cooking apparatus) for cooking by allowing the temperature to rise to the appropriate temperature before heating the food.

Puree: A processing term meaning to cut-down, blend, or process a food until it becomes a thick liquid. The liquid is also called a puree.

Reduce: A method of thickening a sauce or liquid by allowing the water to cook off, and thus, evaporate from the fluid.

Roast: A dry-heat cooking method, usually applied to meats. Roasting is done without a liquid and usually completed in an oven.

Render: Removing fat from meat by cooking, heating, and/or straining the fat from the meat.

Sauté: Cooking method in which a small amount of hot oil is used to heat and brown foods.

Score: To lightly cut the surface of a food in order to tenderize it while cooking.

Sear: Cooking method in which food is quickly browned on all sides before cooking thoroughly. Searing is done to trap flavors and juices.

Shred: Cutting method in which food is taken across a shredding surface to cut small, thin strips. Some foods may be shredded by hand-chopping.

Simmer: To cook foods in liquid that is just below the boiling point.

Steam: Method of cooking in which steam is used to heat food. Steaming may be done using a steaming basket, a steamer, or a pressure-cooker.

Toss: Mixing method in which foods are lightly mixed by a "tossing" or lifting and dropping motion.

Whip: Mixing method, in which food is mixed in a quick and light method to incorporate air into the food. Whipping is often done with a whisk, fork, mixer, or blender, and the cook should use strokes that are fast and follow an up and down pattern.

Zest: The colorful, outer rind of citrus fruits, which is often used to add flavor to sauces, breads, pastries, and other foods. The zest is often grated to remove it from the fruit.

FOOD SUBSTITUTIONS

Common food substitutions include the following:

- Baking powder, 1tsp = ½ tsp cream of tartar plus ¼ tsp baking soda
- Brown sugar (packed), 1c = 1 c granulated sugar plus 1 Tbsp molasses
- Butter = margarine; shortening
- Buttermilk, 1c = 1 Tbsp lemon juice/vinegar per 1c milk; 1c plain yogurt
- Corn syrup, 1c = 1c granulated sugar plus water
- Cornstarch, 1Tbsp (for thickening) = Flour, 1Tbsp
- Cracker crumbs = bread crumbs
- Dried beans, 1lb = 5 c cooked beans
- Granulated Sugar, 1c = 1c brown sugar; 2c powdered sugar
- Milk, 1c = ¼-1/3c dry milk plus 1c water; ½c evaporated milk plus 1c water

*Note: Substitutions may affect quality or taste of finished product.

Food Composition

MACRONUTRIENT AND MICRONUTRIENT

Macronutrient is the term applied to a nutrient that is essential to one's physical health and functioning. Macronutrients must be consumed in large quantities. Fats, proteins, and carbohydrates are macronutrients. Specific macronutrients include: amino acids (such as glutamine, aspartate, tryptophan), monosaturated fats, polysaturated fats, saturated fats, fatty acids, fiber, starch, and sugars. Some minerals are considered macrominerals because they are required in large quantities. Specific macrominerals include: calcium, potassium, magnesium, and sodium.

Micronutrients are minerals and elements that while essential to one's physical health and wellness are needed only in small amounts. The most common (and most commonly deficient) micronutrients include iodine, vitamin A, and iron. Micronutrients are also the source of the many important antioxidants that promote overall health and wellness.

FAT-SOLUBLE VITAMINS

The following are fat-soluble vitamins:

The importance of *vitamin A* in the visual cycle is well documented. One form of vitamin A combines with a protein in the eye to form rhodopsin, which is essential to night vision. The eyes also need vitamin A to maintain mucus-forming cells that lubricate the surface. Vitamin A also helps in immune function, reproductive health and cell development.

Vitamin D, which is also considered a hormone, is essential to the regulation of calcium and bone development. Vitamin D helps the absorption of calcium in the intestine, causes the kidneys to reabsorb calcium, and controls the deposition of calcium in bones.

Vitamin E, which includes a family of compounds called the tocopherols and tocotrienols, acts as one of the body's antioxidants. Vitamin E buffers the assault of free radicals on the body by acting as an electron donor, causing a more stable compound to form.

Vitamin K is essential for the normal function of the body's blood-clotting mechanism. Vitamin K is necessary for the synthesis of several of the body's blood-clotting factors, including prothrombin.

CALCIUM

All cells need calcium to function, and over 99% of calcium in the body works to form and maintain bones and teeth. The role that calcium plays in cellular function is so important that insufficient intake of the mineral will result in decreased bone mass, or osteopenia. Calcium allows for normal blood clotting, acting as a catalyst to the clotting factor prothrombin. Calcium is vital to muscle contraction, allowing protein in the muscles to interact during contraction. Abnormal calcium metabolism can prevent the muscles from relaxing, a condition called tetany. Calcium functions in the transmission of nerve signals by permitting the flow of ions in and out of cells, and also by helping to release neurotransmitters. Finally, calcium plays a role in metabolism by regulating various enzymes, including those that manufacture glycogen.

FACTORS THAT AFFECT THE ABSORPTION OF CALCIUM AND IRON

Calcium is best absorbed in the acidic environment of the duodenum. Vitamin D plays an important role in calcium absorption by stimulating production of calcium binding protein. Calcium is also absorbed through passive diffusion throughout the intestine. Calcium is absorbed only in water-soluble form and usually 70-80% remains unabsorbed and is excreted in waste. The transfer of iron is dependent on a protein carrier synthesized in the liver called transferrin. This protein makes iron available to the cells responsible for heme synthesis. Dietary iron occurs in heme form, found in hemoglobin and myoglobin, and nonheme form, present in plant sources. Gastric acidity increases the availability and absorption of iron from foods. Ascorbic acid increases absorption by forming a compound with iron that is more soluble in the alkaline environment of the small intestine. Lack of gastric acidity or consumption of alkaline products such as antacids decreases iron absorption.

BASAL METABOLIC RATE

Basal metabolism represents the minimum energy expenditure it takes to keep a body at rest alive, so that heartbeat, breathing, temperature maintenance, and other essential functions are maintained. About 40% of the roughly 1400 calories a day needed for survival are used by the brain and liver, 20% by lean muscle mass, and the rest by fat tissue. Lean muscle mass is one of the primary factors in determining one's BMR, so males usually have a higher BMR due to their muscle mass. Aging is associated with a decline in BMR, especially if muscle mass decreases. Physical activity can counteract this by maintaining lean body mass. Febrile patients, trauma patients, and pregnant women have an increased basal metabolism. A low caloric intake can decrease the BMR by as much as 10 to 20% a day, which presents a challenge to individuals following weight loss plans.

POLYSACCHARIDES

Cellulose is a plant fiber that forms the structure of cell walls. The same properties that give structure to plants also contribute to the tough, fibrous texture of fruits and vegetables. This undesirable quality can be lessened in the cooking process. Humans do not possess the ability to break cellulose down, thus the function of this polysaccharide is to add bulk in the diet. *Dextrins* are produced during the breakdown of starch. They have many uses in the food industry, for example the maltodextrin derived from cornstarch so commonly added to many products. Dextrins are easily digested and inexpensive. *Glycogen* is an animal starch with many branches in its structure. More branching in a starch molecule means more sites for enzymes to work on. This makes glycogen very easy to break down, and therefore makes it a good way to store carbohydrates in the body.

HYDROGENATION OF FATS

Hydrogenation contributes to the stability and shelf life of products like pastries, chips, crackers, frosting, and candies. It prevents the fat in the product from weeping oils, so that the frosting on the cookie remains palatable, and it keeps fats solid that would otherwise liquefy at room temperatures, such as margarine. The process of hydrogenation involves converting unsaturated fatty acids to saturated fatty acids by adding hydrogen to the carbons in the fatty acid chain by using high temperatures, a metal catalyst, or hydrogen gas applied under pressure. The result is a structure different from the naturally occurring kinked shape that results from hydrogens on the same side at the double bond. Synthetically hydrogenated fats are called trans fatty acids because the hydrogen molecules are attached to the fatty acid chain in alternating 180-degree fashion, straightening the natural curve of the chain.

BREAKDOWN OF FATS

Fats in the diet are an important part of the body's energy source, even when carbohydrates are present. The liver is the center of lipid metabolism, serving several important functions: to make triglycerides from carbohydrates and proteins, to make other lipids like cholesterol the body needs from triglycerides, to de-saturate fatty acids so that they can be stored in adipose cells, and to break down triglycerides for use as energy. Most fats in the diet are absorbed through the small intestine and enter the lymphatic system. They then travel to the liver and are stored, used immediately for energy, or broken down. Lipoprotein lipase is the enzyme responsible for breaking down triglycerides into fatty acids small enough to pass into human fat cells. Fatty acids are oxidized in the liver to ultimately form acetyl-CoA, which then enters the citric acid cycle with oxaloacetic acid to yield ATP for energy.

ABSORBING VITAMINS A, D, AND B-12

Vitamin A is released from proteins in the stomach. Natural vitamin A in the form of retinyl esters are broken down in the small intestine to form retinol, which are transported in the lymphatic system and then to the liver, where most storage takes place.

SOURCES OF VITAMINS

Vitamin A	Vitamin C	Vitamin E	Calcium	Vitamin D
Liver	Asparagus	Almonds	Dairy products	Fortified milk
Carrots	Broccoli	Hazelnuts	Tofu	Dairy products
Sweet Potato/Yams	Brussels Sprouts	Spinach	Soybeans	Salmon
Butternut Squash	Antelope	Sweet Potatoes	Rhubarb	Herring
Mango	Kiwi	Wheat Germ	Salmon	Sardines
Cantaloupe	Papaya	Avocado	Leafy-green vegetables	Eggs
Apricots	Strawberries	Peanuts	Oysters	Some organ meats
Green leafy	Oranges	Sunflower Seeds		*Sunlight
vegetables	Red Pepper	Vegetable Oils		
Milk				

*Note: Vitamin D aids the absorption of calcium but does not naturally occur in many foods. Sunlight is the best source of Vitamin D, though overexposure to the sun's rays may lead to cancer and other skin diseases. Brief exposure of the hands, face, and arms to the sun is generally sufficient.

When vitamin A is needed in the body it binds with retinol-binding protein and travels from the liver through circulation. Vitamin D is absorbed from the intestine with the aid of bile. Vitamin D is bound to a protein for transport and stored in the liver, skin, bones, and brain. Thiamin is easily absorbed in the first part of the small intestine by active transport, and absorption is inhibited by folate deficiency and alcohol intake. The absorption of riboflavin occurs in the small intestine and is enhanced by the presence of food in the GI tract. The bonds of vitamin B-12 are broken down in the acidic environment of the stomach. However, it is poorly absorbed from the intestine without the presence of the intrinsic factor enzyme.

Principles of Basic and Normal Nutrition

NUTRIENTS/PHYTOCHEMICALS

HORMONES

Hormones that regulate the digestive tract:

- *Gastrin:* Originates in the pyloric region and stimulates the flow of stomach enzymes and acid. Gastrin is produced in greater response to the stimuli of coffee, alcohol, spices, and protein.
- *Gastric inhibitory peptide:* Reduces stomach motility and also inhibits the secretion of stomach acid and enzymes. Fats and proteins stimulate the secretion of this hormone, which originates in the duodenum and jejunum.
- *Cholecystokinin, also referred to as CCK:* Originates in the duodenum and jejunum, and is released especially in response to the presence of fat and protein in the duodenum. This hormone causes the gallbladder to contract, releasing bile into the duodenum. CCK also causes the release of enzyme-rich pancreatic juices and bicarbonate-rich pancreatic juices.

- *Secretin*: Functions by stimulating the secretion of thin bicarbonate-rich pancreatic juice, offering a buffering effect, and it also reduces stomach motility. Secretin is stimulated by the acidic substance chyme entering the stomach. This hormone originates in the duodenum and the jejunum.

BLOOD SUGAR CONTROL

Blood sugar is regulated primarily by the endocrine pancreas through the action of insulin and glucagon, which exert opposing influences in the body. Insulin is released by the beta cells of the pancreas in response to the presence of elevated blood sugar after eating. Insulin increases the synthesis of glycogen in the liver and also stimulates glucose to move from the bloodstream into muscle and fat cells, thereby lowering blood sugar levels and promoting glucose storage. A few hours after eating, when glucose levels begin to fall, glucagon is produced by alpha cells in the pancreas. This hormone elevates blood sugar level by prompting glycogen breakdown in the liver. Epinephrine is a powerful blood sugar stimulant, but it is secreted by the adrenal medulla. Its role is also to stimulate a breakdown of glycogen in the liver and therefore elevate glucose in the bloodstream.

THYROXINE, GLUCOCORTICOIDS, AND ADRENOCORTICOTROPIC

Thyroxine, which is manufactured by the follicular cells of the thyroid, plays a role in carbohydrate metabolism and protein metabolism. Patients with hypothyroidism may see their basal metabolic rate fall from 30 to 50%. Thyroxine affects protein metabolism by increasing the rate of metabolism in all cells.

Glucocorticoids, such as cortisol, raise blood glucose levels by stimulating gluconeogenesis. These hormones counteract the effects of insulin by reducing glucose use in the body and increasing the rate at which protein is turned into glucose.

ACTH is secreted from the pituitary gland, and works to reduce the effects of glucose by stimulating the adrenal cortex to grow and release glucocorticoids. This hormone is part of the neuroendocrine response and is stimulated by stress, allowing the body to mobilize resources, such as amino acids stored in the muscle, to be used as energy.

BASIC HUMAN PHYSIOLOGY

EXERCISE

Water functions in the body to transport nutrients and waste products to and from cells, and allows the body to maintain temperature control. The water lost during exercise comes from increased respiration and sweating. Fluid lost from sweat comes from the blood volume, so dehydration can impair cardiovascular functioning. Fluids should be consumed in adequate amounts to maintain pre-exercise weight. The first source of energy for exercising muscles is *glycogen* stored in the muscle. When that is exhausted, the liver maintains the glucose supply via gluconeogenesis and glycogenolysis. The liver can maintain blood glucose for extended periods this way, but depletion can occur after long distance events. After heavy training it can take up to 24 hours to renew glycogen stores.

Protein is more important in terms of functioning as an energy source to the athlete than for building muscle. The amount of protein needed to build new muscle is met by the average diet, and the RDA for protein for athletes is the same as for the general population.

CONVERTING PROTEIN

Proteins fulfill a major structural role in the body in the building and maintenance of tissues. They also play a role in the formation of hormones, enzymes, and antibodies. Proteins consist of an amino group and a carboxyl group joined to a carbon atom. The basic protein structure has a free carboxyl group at one end and a free amino group at the other. More amino acids can join at either end to form different proteins. When proteins are used for energy, the liver detaches the amino groups and the carbon skeletons converted into glucose, ketone bodies, or other substances that can enter the citric acid cycle and produce ATP. Before protein can be used as a structural component in the body all of the essential amino acids must be available. The body can then form the specific proteins it needs under the control of DNA, with energy from ATP driving the process.

VALVES

The *upper and lower esophageal sphincters* control the flow of food through the esophagus. The lower esophageal sphincter plays an important role in preventing heartburn, as it stops food from flowing from the stomach back into the esophagus. The *pyloric sphincter,* located at the base of the stomach, allows the acidic contents of the stomach to enter the small intestine a few milliliters at a time. The *sphincter of Oddi,* located at the end of the gallbladder, relaxes in response to the hormone Cholecystokinin, allowing bile to enter the duodenum. The *ileocecal valve*, located at the end of the small intestine, prevents the bacteria laden contents of the large intestine from entering the small intestine. At the end of the rectum are two *anal* sphincters, which are under voluntary control and allow for the release of fecal waste.

PROCESS OF PERISTALSIS

Peristalsis is a series of coordinated muscular movements that propel food from the esophagus to the anus. A circular group of muscles constricts and relaxes behind and in front of the ingested food, allowing it to move down the GI tract. A second group of muscles that runs lengthwise along the GI tract then contract, which makes the GI tract shorter. This coordinated squeezing and shortening moves the food through the esophagus in two main waves to the stomach, where the peristalsis action functions in a mixing and grinding fashion as frequently as three times a minute. The small intestine has rapid peristalsis movements, which function more to mix the chyme rather than to move the food along. The colon features less frequent movements, employing occasional large waves that coordinate contraction along the length of the colon to help produce bowel movements.

TYPES OF ABSORPTION

The four basic types of absorption processes used in the small intestine:

- *Passive absorption*: Requires no carrier molecules or energy in order for the nutrient to pass through the wall of the intestine. The substance must be present in a higher concentration in the lumen of the small intestine than in the absorptive cells for this to take place.
- *Active absorption:* Uses energy to pump the nutrient, such as amino acids, into the intestine's villi. This process requires the use of ATP as the driving energy force.
- *Facilitated absorption:* Uses a carrier molecule to transport the nutrients from the lumen of the intestine into the absorptive cells, but no energy is needed.
- *Phagocytosis:* Means the absorptive cell actually surrounds and engulfs the nutrient. Breast milk antibodies ingested by infants are absorbed this way.

LARGE INTESTINE

While the small intestine is the major site for nutrient absorption, the large intestine functions to prepare the last undigested remnants to be excreted as feces. The ingested foodstuffs that eventually reach the colon consist mostly of water, some minerals, and some plant fibers and starches. Only a very small percentage of carbohydrate, protein, and fat remain. The colon does function to absorb some water, although nearly 90% has already been absorbed by the small intestine. The colon absorbs vitamin K, sodium, and potassium along the first half. By the time the stool reaches the descending colon, peristaltic waves push the mass toward the rectum, and the urge to eliminate stimulates the anal sphincters to relax.

GLYCOLYSIS PATHWAY

The function of the glycolysis pathway is to break down glucose. Not only does the process break down single sugars for the body to use as energy, it also provides the building blocks the body needs to help form essential compounds like glycerol for triglyceride formation. Glucose is stored as glycogen in the liver and muscle cells, and the net result of the glycolytic pathway is to take this six-carbon form of glucose and break it down into two molecules of pyruvate. During this process each molecule of glucose has the potential to create 36 to 38 ATP molecules, either by yielding NADH, a potential form of energy, or ATP, a source of energy the body can use immediately.

NUTRIENT NEEDS AT VARIOUS STAGES
EFFECTS OF AGING

Aging takes its toll on all of the body's systems, not least of which is the gastrointestinal system. Changes may occur in the mouth, which may include decreased production of saliva, changes in olfactory abilities, including the ability to taste, and changes in the teeth, gums, and palates. These changes may result in difficulties tasting, chewing, and swallowing food. Additionally, the gastrointestinal tract's ability to move food through via peristalsis may be impaired in the esophagus and stomach, which may further reduce one's ability to swallow, cause heartburn, constipation, and other problems processing and metabolizing food. Other changes, including reduced blood flow to the gastrointestinal tract and liver may result in additional discomfort as the body's ability to process food is hindered.

DRI

Dietary Reference Intakes (DRI) are meant to replace the Recommended Dietary Allowances that have long provided reference values to help people know how much of what nutrient they should be getting in an adequate diet. Rather than providing one catchall value for all individuals, this reference includes the estimated average requirement (EAR), adequate intake (AI), and tolerable upper intake levels (UL). While the RDA shared values that would meet the nutritional needs of most individuals when consumed daily, DRI shares goals that are meant to be achieved over time. EAR provides the intake that would meet the needs of half the population using median, rather than average to determine which 50% is included in the reference group. If not enough data is available to determine EAR, then AI is an estimate that assumes an adequate value in healthy people. UL levels should not be exceeded, or nutrient toxicity may occur.

DIETARY GUIDELINES FOR AMERICANS

Every five years, the USDA and the HHS publish a new set of Dietary Guidelines to provide advice about how good nutrition can help children over the age of two and adults achieve good health and reduce their risk for chronic diseases. These guidelines are the basis for federal food and nutrition programs such as WIC and the food stamp program. The guidelines also provide the basis for the consumer-friendly My Pyramid food guidance system. The focus areas in the 2005 report look at the challenges of ingesting adequate nutrients within calorie needs; maintaining ideal weight; getting enough physical activity; which food groups are to be encouraged; guidelines for the intake of carbohydrate, fats, sodium, and potassium; moderation in alcohol consumption; and food borne illness prevention techniques. The recent report offers more specificity for proportions in that recommended amounts are described in cups or ounces rather than the ambiguous term "servings."

CHILDHOOD NUTRITIONAL REQUIREMENTS

Children need extra energy and nutrients in relation to their size because they are growing and developing bones, muscle, and blood. Children also have higher basal metabolic rates, increasing their need for calories even at rest. Children triple their birth weight in the first year of life, and increase their length by 50%. Growth slows until adolescence, when the child will gain 20% of his or her adult height and 50% of his or her adult weight. Protein intake should range from 1.2 grams per kg in early childhood to 1 gram per kg in late childhood. Protein deficiency in children is rarely a problem in the U.S. because of the abundance of protein-rich foods. Iron deficiency anemia is common in preschool aged children because the rapid rate of growth may not be supported by enough iron-rich foods in the diet. Calcium is essential for mineralization and maintenance of growing bones. Vitamin D is necessary for proper calcium absorption, and may be found in fortified milk.

PALATABILITY OF FOOD

Food palatability is determined by at least four of a human's five senses: taste, smell, sight, and touch. The physical appearance and texture of a menu item is paramount to the presentation of the food. If a menu item is visually unappealing, one is less likely to eat it. Furthermore, textures of food—both on the plate and on the palate—may or may not be appealing to the consumer. Failure to properly prepare food often results in unappetizing appearance, texture, and smell. Smell is quite possibly the most involved of the senses as it plays a role in both the initial response to the presented menu item as well as the actual flavor of the food. Food flavor is received by the human anatomy through a marriage of both taste and aroma. The aroma of food is received by the olfactory receptors in the nasal passage and blended with the messages received and transmitted by the taste buds on the tongue. This marriage of signals is then communicated to the brain, which is able to decipher and deliver a flavor response.

Nutrition Care for Individuals and Groups

Screening and Assessment

NUTRITION ASSESSMENTS

A nutritional assessment is performed to determine the nutritional needs and habits of a client. The assessment may be essential to finding and understanding dietary deficiencies or excesses as well as to formulation of a nutritional plan for a client. Nutritional assessments most often incorporate a variety of data, which assess physical and biochemical traits, dietary habits, and psychosocial well-being. Physical traits are evaluated through the use of anthropometric measurements, including height, weight, and body mass index, among others. Biochemical tests are used to assess protein, vitamin, and mineral deficiencies. Psychosocial assessments help the practitioner determine whether depression, lack of social interaction, or other factors may influence a client's dietary habits. When performing and evaluating a nutritional assessment, it is imperative that all parts of the assessment are considered. Daily dietary changes, life stresses, hydration levels, and medical therapies may all skew individual tests results and clinical presentation.

CLINICAL DATA

Clinical data help round out the nutritional assessment picture. Such data may include medical and treatment histories as well as any current treatment information. Life stresses, medical treatments, including surgeries, therapies, and pharmaceutical interventions, over-the-counter medicine use, and daily routine may all affect one's nutritional status. Absorption of key nutrients is frequently impeded or altered by drug therapies and life stresses. As with all parts of the nutritional assessment, the clinical data must be evaluated by a professional and in accordance to information gleaned from other data, such as anthropometric measurements, biochemical tests, diet journal, and patient history.

ASSESSMENT FORMS

The nutritional assessment form is called the Minimum Data Set (MDS). MDS is a patient overview/history that is included in the medical chart. The MDS assesses every aspect (physical, social, psychological, emotional, et cetera) of a patient's status. Included in the MDS is a brief overview (Section AC) followed by a lengthy listing of questions regarding a patient's history. In addition to the questions regarding a patient's eating patterns in Section AC, an in-depth assessment of oral and nutritional health appears in Section K. That assessment includes questions regarding intake, weight gain or loss, ability to taste, problems chewing or swallowing, and the use of feeding devices such as tube and intravenous feeding supplements.

MEDICAL CHARTS

Medical charts must be maintained with the highest regard to precision and accuracy. Because many medical personnel may be accessing the chart on a daily basis, it is important that documents be placed in the correct section of the medical record and that notes are clearly and legibly written. Dietary information is most often found in the dietary section and/or progress notes section of a medical chart. Additionally, the nutritional assessment form, called the minimum data set, is also an important document to reference. Be careful to document all notes, progress reports, and recommendations accurately and legibly, always in blue or black (preferred) ink. When a change is necessary, using an ink pen, draw a single line through the text. Do not scribble or completely block out the previously written notes. Some facilities also require that all revisions be initialed.

SPECIFIC ASSESSMENTS

TRICEPS SKIN FOLD, WAIST/HIP RATION, ARM MUSCLE AREA, AND BODY MASS INDEX

Triceps skin fold is an anthropometric measurement that can be used to estimate an individual's body fat. A device called a caliper is used to pinch the skin and underlying fatty tissue without disturbing the muscle layer.

Waist to hip ratio is indicative of the distribution of abdominal fat deposits. A WHR of greater than 1.0 in men or .8 in women indicates that the individual is at a higher risk for cardiovascular disease and diabetes.

Arm muscle is an important measurement used in children to assess whether the child has an adequate skeletal muscle mass. If a growing child is not receiving enough carbohydrates in the diet, protein that would otherwise be used to build muscle mass is burned as energy.

Body mass index is a formula that can be used to screen for the presence of excess adipose tissue, which may cause weight related problems. The formula is weight (kg) / [height (m)]^2.

NUTRITIONAL ASSESSMENT OF POPULATIONS

The rationale for the Nutritional Assessment of Populations is to gain an understanding of the biological, cultural, and environmental factors that contribute or take away from the nutritional status of communities determined to be at risk. The program also seeks to assess how well existing programs are serving the health needs of the community and how problem areas identified in the assessment process can be addressed so that health is enhanced. Research relies on a variety of epidemiologic and anthropologic methods applied to areas that are deemed to be socially or economically depressed. The tools that serve as sources of information include assessment of growth and physical activity of the population; the existence and utilization of social services such as WIC, school foodservice programs, and free health clinics; analysis of socioeconomic factors coming from data on public housing usage or census data; and demographics, morbidity, and mortality rates.

NSI AND THE ELDERLY

The Nutrition Screening Initiative (NSI) helps elderly individuals in the U.S. at risk for compromised nutritional status by identifying those at risk due to their financial, social, or functional status. It also considers one's access to food. The "DETERMINE" acronym can be used to describe the list of factors health professionals or social service agencies look at when determining risk:

> D = Disease
> E = Eating Poorly
> T = Tooth loss or mouth pain
> E = Economic hardship
> R = Reduced social contact
> M = Multiple medications
> I = Involuntary weight loss or gain
> N = Needs assistance in self care
> E = Elder years above 80

The benefits of the screening tool include ease of use and ability to identify patients in need of more comprehensive screening. Limitations include the tool's dependency on patient's ability or willingness to cooperate.

NATIVE AMERICAN AND ALASKAN NATIVE POPULATIONS

As Native Americans and Alaskan natives have traded traditional foods such as deer meat and buffalo for foods high in calories and saturated fat like hamburger and fast foods, the population has seen an obesity epidemic. Accompanying obesity-related diseases such as diabetes, heart disease, and hypertension have risen accordingly. Limited food availability on reservations can also contribute to intake patterns. Processed meats and sugar-sweetened drinks are popular mainstays in many reservation markets, while fresh produce is often limited. Baby bottle tooth decay is another nutritional problem that affects a large number of both Native Americans and Alaskan Natives. Prolonged bottle use is common and sugar-sweetened drinks are offered throughout the day. Although fluoridated water is available, drinking water may be obtained from rainwater or wells, with drinking water saved for other household uses. Native Americans and Alaskan natives have higher rates of alcohol abuse, which contributes to the malabsorption of several nutrients, as well as liver disease.

MIGRANTS AND HOMELESS INDIVIDUALS

The lifestyle of migrants provides several challenges for nutritional assessment and intervention. The families move from season to season, making continuity of care difficult. The public health systems they utilize do not communicate across communities, so medical records and other health documents need to be transported with the patient. Language and cultural barriers can interfere with nutrition education and counseling. Nutrition education may focus on issues specific to the group, such as prenatal care and diabetes services. Individuals experiencing homelessness frequently have mental health issues that interfere with their ability to seek social services available to them. Emergency food programs may not provide balanced nutrition, and many programs are ill-equipped to meet the needs of infants and children. Homeless families who qualify for WIC may not have the transportation to reach the provider. For homeless individuals who do not routinely use shelters, storage and proper preparation of food is an issue.

DIET HISTORY

A diet history is essential to determining the current nutritional habits of a client and developing an ongoing nutritional plan for the individual(s). A diet history should include information about the client's daily intake, disabilities and/or conditions that may impede the client's ability to consume various types of food, ethnic and cultural influences (flavoring, food staples, prohibited foods), and religious restrictions (meals must be kosher, does not eat meat, seasonal food restrictions, etc.). Additionally, it is important to inquire about allergies, drug therapies (some foods may interfere with drug absorption and/or pharmaceuticals may alter tastes), sense of taste and smell, and appetite. When taking a diet history, it may be helpful to employ recording methods such as utilizing a 3-day food record, administering a food frequency questionnaire, and interviewing the client (as well as his/her caretaker, if applicable).

When interviewing, it is important to do so in a manner that is neither leading nor intimidating to the client. If the client is not a native English speaker, arrange for a translator to assist with the interview. Likewise, if the client is unable to communicate and/or is suffering from memory loss/dementia, it is advisable to have a family member or other caretaker present at the interview. When asking questions, be aware of phrasing so as to avoid leading a client to answer in a manner that would appease the interviewer. For example, instead of asking, "You don't eat dessert at every meal, do you?" You may ask, "Approximately how many servings of sweets (to include cookies, cakes, puddings, pies, etc.) do you eat daily?" Finally, watch for nonverbal cues from the client. Consistent head-nodding may indicate that the individual does not fully understand the question or language used. Lack of eye contact and focus may be a sign that the client is not alert or that he/she may be confused.

CHILDREN AND PREGNANT WOMEN

The CDC has two major programs in place to monitor the health and nutritional status of low-income women, infants, and children. The Pediatric Nutrition Surveillance System (PedNSS) uses data from the Women, Infants, and Children program (WIC), the Early and Periodic Screening, Diagnosis, and Treatment (EPSDT) Program, and the Title V Maternal and Child Health Program. Data is analyzed to discover trends in birth weight, anemia, breastfeeding, stature, and other nutrition-related indicators. The goal of the program is to use this surveillance data to implement and evaluate existing health programs and formulate public policy. The Pregnancy Nutrition Surveillance System (PNSS) looks at maternal health and nutritional status of low-income women, but is more concerned with maternal nutrition as it relates to the outcome of the infant. Data on maternal weight gain, prenatal vitamin intake, and pregnancy-related complications like diabetes are evaluated in the context of birth outcomes like preterm delivery and low birth weight. Results are used to guide public health policy.

Diagnosis

DIABETES

Diabetes is a disease in which the pancreas is not able to effectively regulate insulin production, and, therefore, the body's cells do not receive needed amounts of glucose. When an individual consumes carbohydrates, those carbohydrates are broken down into glucose, which immediately enters the bloodstream. In a correctly functioning body, the pancreas then produces insulin, which aids in the cells' absorption of glucose. However, in patients with diabetes, the insulin production is either insufficient or dysfunctional and the glucose is unable to reach the cells.

There are two long-term forms of diabetes. Type 1 Diabetes (more commonly known as juvenile-onset or insulin-dependent diabetes) occurs when the insulin-production system is permanently disabled. On the other hand, Type 2 Diabetes develops gradually and is often the result of poor diet and exercise habits. In this type, the cells no longer respond to insulin, and thus, the production of insulin begins to fail.

If not properly treated and managed, diabetes can lead to many long-term health issues, including blindness, heart disease, stroke, foot and leg problems, and others.

HOW DIABETES MAY AFFECT ONE'S DIETARY NEEDS

Diets designed specifically for diabetic patients should be formulated to promote healthy blood glucose, cholesterol, and blood pressure levels. Because diabetes is directly related to the body's ability to process, store, and utilize carbohydrates, -it is important to monitor carbohydrate intake. While a well-balanced diet that follows the guidelines set forth in MyPlate is generally adequate for a patient with diabetes, many dietitians recommend an exchange diet, which allows the patient relative dietary freedom while still monitoring carbohydrate (sugar and starch) intake. Sugars may be substituted for starches in the exchange diet; however, doing so diminishes the nutritional value of the entire meal. Additionally, artificial sweeteners do not seem to have an effect on blood glucose. In addition to closely monitoring carbohydrate consumption, patients with diabetes should aim to eat a heart-healthy diet. Because of their increased risk for heart disease, avoiding trans and saturated fats as well as foods with high cholesterol content is advisable.

RECOMMENDATIONS FOR PROTEIN, FAT, AND CARBOHYDRATE INTAKE

Protein needs of the diabetic patient should be calculated in a similar way to the protein needs of the general population, varying from .8g/kg for adults to somewhere between 1-2.2 g/kg for infants and children. This results in protein providing between 15-20% of total energy intake. Some research suggests that keeping the protein intake on the lower end of the spectrum, between 12-15% of total energy intake, can delay kidney disease. To help guard against the vascular disease common in diabetics, fat should make up less than 30% of total energy intake, and cholesterol intake should stay under 300 mg/day. Saturated fats should account for less than 10% of lipids in the diet.

Protein	Phosphorus	Sodium
Meat	Dairy Products	Table Salts
Poultry	Dried beans	Processed Cheese
Seafood	Dried Peas	Canned/Prepared Meals
Dairy Products	Soft Drinks	Pickled Foods
Eggs	Nuts	Fast Food
Other Animal Products	Peanut Butter	Cured Meats

The recommended amount of carbohydrate in the diet can vary depending on the patient's blood glucose response, but usually ranges from 55-60%. Research suggests that providing ~10% of energy in the form of monounsaturated fats instead of carbohydrates results in a more favorable lipid profile for diabetics.

KIDNEY DISEASE

Kidney disease affects the body's ability to process and eliminate waste and extraneous fluid from the body and blood stream. Dietary changes may help in the management of the disease. The most common dietary changes implemented in individuals with kidney disease include controlling the amount of protein and limiting phosphorus and sodium intake. Note the lists below, which identify foods with high levels of protein, phosphorus, and sodium.

Clients with kidney disease should also avoid multivitamins as the body has a difficult time breaking down some vitamins and minerals.

CANCER

Patients with cancer often suffer from a myriad of symptoms, which may affect their diets. Some common symptoms of cancer and side effects of treatment include fatigue, altered sense of taste and smell, nausea, vomiting, diarrhea, constipation, dry, sore mouth, and others. It is important that cancer patients receive a well-balanced diet, rich in vitamins and minerals. Additionally, because of their generally weakened immune system, patients with cancer should avoid raw, undercooked, and unpasteurized foods, all of which are more susceptible to bacteria. Frequently, clients with cancer will also be advised to follow a high-calorie diet, which provides greater energy to assist in combating fatigue. Employ strategies, such as adding additional sugar/sweetener, to enhance the flavors of the food and, in turn, make mealtime a more enjoyable experience.

HEART DISEASE

Patients with cardiovascular disease may suffer from a variety of ailments, to include high blood pressure and cholesterol levels, high risk of stroke, heart attack, and more. Therefore, dietary modification is an effective way to prevent and treat patients with heart disease. Common recommendations include implementing a low-sodium (less than 2300 mg/day), low-cholesterol diet (less than 300 mg/day), eliminating trans fats by eliminating partially hydrogenated vegetable oils and fried foods, reducing sugar intake, and consuming only the calories needed to meet one's daily energy requirements. Additionally, it is advisable for patients at-risk or suffering from heart disease to increase their fruit and vegetable intake, maximizing vitamin, mineral, and antioxidant consumption, as well as to eat a diet high in fiber.

PREGNANCY

Vitamin D is essential in skeletal formation in the fetus and for the metabolism of calcium. Calcium metabolism increases during pregnancy, so the recommended dietary allowance (RDA) for vitamin D doubles from 5 to 10 micrograms a day. This increase may be satisfied by regular sunlight exposure, increasing one's consumption of vitamin D milk, or via supplementation. Folate plays an important role in the synthesis of nucleic acids, and is therefore necessary to DNA formation. Beginning one's pregnancy with an adequate store of folic acid is important in reducing certain birth defects, such as spinal malformations. The RDA for folate increases from 180 micrograms for adult females to 400 micrograms, which ideally should begin before conception. Red blood cell formation increases dramatically during pregnancy, so the RDA for iron doubles from 15 to 30 milligrams a day. Although it remains important to seek out iron-rich foods such as red meat or spinach, supplementation is usually necessary to provide adequate amounts to prevent such problems as premature delivery and low birth weight.

COMMON DIETARY MODIFICATIONS

Pregnant women should be encouraged to eat a healthy, balanced diet packed with fruits, vegetables, whole grains, protein, and dairy products. Typically, during her pregnancy, a healthy woman should consume between 200 and 400 more healthy calories per day. Depending on pre-pregnancy weight, caloric consumption may be more or less. Additionally, pregnant women have higher demands for vitamins and minerals, especially, folic acid, calcium, and iron. Pregnancy also demands large fluid stores in a woman's body; therefore, pregnant woman should consume at least eight glasses (more with physical activity) of water per day. In addition to increasing nutrients, pregnant women should avoid some foods. Those foods include alcohol and some types of seafood with generally high mercury levels, namely, shark, swordfish, mackerel, or tilefish.

SUPPLEMENT A PREGNANT WOMAN'S DIET

Pregnant women should consume additional folic acid and calcium in their diet. The following are foods that are rich in calcium and folate.

Folic Acid	Calcium
Enriched cereals	Calcium-fortified juices
Enriched grains	Calcium-fortified cereals
Legumes	Dairy products
Black beans	Green leafy vegetables
Spinach	Almonds
Asparagus	Salmon
Green leafy vegetables	Tofu
Lentils	Rhubarb
Pinto beans	Beans

THE ELDERLY

With age the senses of taste, sight, and smell diminish, which adversely affects food intake. Medications commonly taken by elderly people can change the taste of food or give food a metallic taste. Impaired function of the gastrointestinal tract can affect nutritional status in several ways. Tooth decay or ill-fitting dentures may interfere with mastication, forcing individuals to give up foods they previously enjoyed. Diminished salivary function due to normal aging or medications also interferes with mastication and swallowing. The large intestine exhibits decreased motility, leading to constipation, which can inhibit appetite. Dementia or depression found in some elderly people may contribute to poor nutritional status, especially if the person lives in isolation. The inability to shop for or prepare food can be one of the leading reasons elderly individuals enter a nursing home. Many senior citizens also struggle with financial difficulties when they stop working. Although two-thirds of these individuals may qualify for the Food Stamp program, less than half use it.

FLUIDS

Symptoms of dehydration include dry mouth, tongue and mucous membranes, decreased urination, sunken eyes, cheeks or abdomen, confusion, light-headedness, dizziness, disorientation, dry skin, fatigue, irritability, thirst, and weight loss, among others. It is recommended that humans consume a minimum 30 milliliters of fluid per kilogram body weight, daily. Thus, the daily recommended fluid intake for a woman weighing 135 lbs is calculated as follows:

Convert pounds to kilograms: 135 lbs x 0.454 kg/lb = 61.29 kg

Daily recommended fluid intake: 61.29 kg x 30 mL/kg = 1838.7 mL

IRON DEFICIENCY

Iron deficiency is best combated by introducing or increasing iron-rich foods in one's diet. Additionally, consumption of Vitamin C rich foods will enhance the absorption of non-heme iron. Iron-rich foods include:

Heme Iron Sources	Non-Heme Iron Sources
Clams	Fortified cereals
Oysters	Soybeans
Shrimp	Squash
Organ Meats	Pumpkin
Beef	Various Beans
Duck	Tomato Products
Lamb	Prune Juice
	Molasses

Iron deficiency can occur for a variety of reasons. Most commonly, individuals experiencing rapid growth (especially infants, children under five years of age, and pubescent females), pregnant women, and those who have lost large amounts of blood (through normal processes such as menstruation, infection or disease, or blood donation, for example) experience iron deficiency. Additionally, individuals who do not eat a healthy diet may also suffer from iron deficiency. Symptoms of an iron deficiency include tiredness/fatigue, slowed development, inability to regulate or maintain body temperature, and impaired immune system functioning, among others.

PRESSURE ULCERS

Pressure ulcers, also known as pressure sores, bed sores, decubitus ulcers, and ischemic ulcers, occur when pressure is placed on one part of the body for too long, without repositioning. Essentially, layers of dermis gradually breakdown from unrelenting pressure to cause open wounds that vary in severity from a reddened area on the skin to an ulcer that has damaged muscle, bone, tendon, and other tissue. Causes of pressure sores include immobility, incontinence (moisture can contribute to tissue breakdown), malnourishment, diabetes and/or circulation problems. Therefore, these sores may be warning signs of malnourishment, in which a balanced, substantial diet needs to be introduced and/or other diseases, such as diabetes, in which other dietary action should also be taken.

ANOREXIA NERVOSA

Anorexia nervosa is a psychiatric disorder in which patients refuse to eat in order to achieve a certain body image. Though individuals suffering from anorexia may literally be starving, the individual most often sees himself/herself as overweight. Anorexia nervosa causes extreme malnourishment and may present via symptoms such as weight loss, sunken eyes, protruding skeletal structure, amenorrhea, constipation, fatigue, low energy, downy hair on the face and neck, and other symptoms. Therapy focusing on behavior modification is essential to recovery from anorexia. Primary dietary concerns are to address malnourishment and introduce healthy eating habits. The diet gradually increases caloric consumption and may aim for more than three meals per day.

BULIMIA NERVOSA

Bulimia is an eating disorder characterized by binging and purging. Purging may be achieved by vomiting or taking laxatives. Bulimia drains the body of all nutrients and electrolytes and causes various digestive tract problems resulting from the constant strain on the system from purging. Bulimia further affects nearly every body system including the cardiac, endocrine, and nervous systems. As with anorexia, behavioral therapy is the recommended treatment. Healthy dietary habits should be introduced and malnourishment immediately addressed. A diet that gradually increases caloric consumption should be prescribed.

CELIAC DISEASE

Celiac disease attacks the small intestine and creates sensitivity to gluten. Gluten is found in wheat, barley, and rye products. Additionally, many products are produced in factories that also manufacture gluten-containing products. Thus, individuals with celiac disease must search for "gluten-free" products. "Gluten-free" products may include any product that does not have the opportunity to come in contact with gluten and extends beyond pastas, breads, and flours. Dietary substitutions for foods containing gluten include soy, rice, potato, nuts, legumes, tapioca, corn, flax seed, and buckwheat. Many vitamins, supplements, and pharmaceuticals also contain gluten. Advise clients to check with their pharmacist before taking any medicines.

GASTROINTESTINAL ULCER

Gastric ulcers are caused by factors leading to impairment of the mucosal barrier, allowing stomach acid to enter the gastric tissue where erosion and eventual ulceration can occur. One cause of this process can be a malfunction of the pyloric sphincter, which allows the alkaline contents of the duodenum to back up into the stomach, where the base content of the fluid acts to lower the mucosal defense. Taking NSAID drugs and infection with the H. pylori bacteria also increases the risk of ulcer development.

Drugs commonly used to treat gastric ulcers include antacids, which neutralize gastric acids; Cimetidine (Tagamet), which inhibits acid secretion; and Sucralfate, which coats and protects the ulcer site. Nutritional care focuses on patient comfort, neutralization of stomach acids, and maintenance of healthy gastric mucosa. Most foods can be allowed as tolerated. Alcohol in high amounts is damaging to the mucosa. Pepper and spicy foods may stimulate acid secretion and can irritate the stomach lining.

DUMPING SYNDROME

Dumping syndrome is a response to the presence of excess amounts of undigested food in the jejunum. When patients have a large amount of the stomach surgically removed and resume a normal diet, the food can pass in large amounts into the jejunum instead of the normal process of gradually passing in small amounts. When the ingested food is broken down rapidly the contents of the intestine can become hypertonic. The body seeks to achieve osmotic balance by drawing water from the plasma to dilute the contents, leading to decrease in blood volume. This causes sweating, weakness, and rapid heartbeat. The digested carbohydrates then rapidly enter the blood stream and cause elevated blood glucose, which triggers overproduction of insulin and subsequent hypoglycemia. Simple carbohydrates, which are hydrolyzed quickly, should be limited. Proteins and fats are better tolerated. Patients with severe dumping may only take liquids between meals, to avoid overwhelming the jejunum.

DIVERTICULAR DISEASES

Diverticulosis is a disease of the large intestine in which pouches collect in the wall of the colon. These pouches may develop as a result of high intracolonic pressure due to a low fiber diet or the reduction of strength of the muscle wall in the colon. The incidence of the disease is increased in elderly populations. Diverticulitis occurs when fecal matter accumulates in the herniations of patients with diverticulosis. This can lead to infection, inflammation, ulceration, and even rupture of the colon wall. It was once believed that adherence to a low fiber diet eased the symptoms of diverticular diseases. It is now understood that high fiber diets increase the movement of waste through the colon and decrease intracolonic pressure, relieving symptoms. For those patients experiencing a flare-up of diverticulitis, a low-residue diet can be followed, gradually introducing high fiber foods as tolerated.

CROHN'S AND ULCERATIVE COLITIS

Crohn's disease is a chronic, progressive disease involving long segments of the large or small intestine with inflammation from the mucosa to the serosa. Ulcerative colitis involves the rectum with possible lower colon involvement, while the right colon and small intestine remain unaffected. Symptoms are similar for both disorders: gradual onset of diarrhea, abdominal pain, weight loss, and blood or pus in the stool. Maintaining fluid and electrolyte balance is important in managing acute flare-ups for both diseases. Surgical intervention, including partial or total removal of the diseased colon may be necessary in severe cases. Patients with inflammatory bowel diseases may be malnourished from recurrent diarrhea and reduced intake caused from pain and fear of eating. Carbohydrate and protein content should be high to restore good nutritional status in those with reduced intake. Vitamin supplementation with iron, vitamin B-12, and folate may be necessary to counteract the effects of malabsorption and blood loss.

ADVERSE EFFECTS OF MEDICATIONS

Bleeding in the GI tract is a common side effect of aspirin, and this causes the body to lose iron even in the absence of obvious symptoms such as blood in the stool. Aspirin can also decrease the uptake of ascorbic acid and alter the distribution of ascorbic acid in the body, leading to decreased amounts in the body and increased excretion in the urine. Diuretics such as thiazide can increase bone resorption or increase intestinal calcium absorption, resulting in the excretion of potassium, sodium, and magnesium through the urine. Corticosteroids can increase protein breakdown, decrease calcium absorption, and decrease protein synthesis. The result can be decreased bone formation, increased excretion of potassium and nitrogen, and increased need for vitamin D. The antidepressant lithium carbonate can cause changes in sodium distribution in the body or excessive excretion. MAOI drugs can increase the appetite, leading to weight gain.

DIARRHEA IN INFANTS AND CHILDREN

Diarrhea is an abnormality of excretion that occurs when stools are frequent and high in liquid content. It is also characterized by an excessive loss of electrolytes, especially sodium and potassium, which can lead to dangerous complications in children. Diarrhea can be the result of the rapid passing of small intestinal contents, preventing the action of digestive enzymes and disallowing for the absorptive action of fluid and nutrients. Diarrhea can also result from changes in the intestinal mucosa.

Diarrhea is a symptom of a disease process rather than a disease in itself, so treatment should aim to manage the underlying disorder. Acute diarrhea can become serious quickly in infants and young children, as their small body mass increases their susceptibility to dehydration and electrolyte imbalances. Aggressive replacement of fluids and electrolytes should be given in the form of an oral rehydration solution. The glucose electrolyte solution recommended by the World Health Organization is composed of specified amounts of glucose, sodium, potassium, chloride, and bicarbonate in a water solution.

STEATORRHEA

Most diseases of malabsorption cause steatorrhea, a condition characterized by the presence of undigested fat in the stool. Regular stools contain two to five grams of fat; however, the stools of patients with steatorrhea may contain up to 60 grams of fat. Diagnosis can be made by keeping a food diary and analyzing the fat content of stools over a 72-hour period, focusing on the ratio of ingested fat to stool fat. Treatment should be tailored according to the underlying condition. Disease processes associated with malabsorption include inadequate digestion, bile salt deficiency, mucosal cell damage, inflammatory disorders, and malfunctions of the intestine's lymphatic system. Weight loss in patients due to fat loss may be countered with increased energy intake in the diet from carbohydrates and protein. Reduced absorption of vitamins and minerals due to the lack of fat as a transport mechanism can be problematic. Supplementation of calcium, iron, zinc, magnesium, and fat-soluble vitamins may be required.

SHORT BOWEL SYNDROME

The small or large intestine may need to be surgically resected for a variety of reasons. Removal of more than two-thirds of the small intestine is sometimes necessary in the treatment of cancer, Crohn's disease, radiation damage, or bowel obstruction, resulting in problems collectively referred to as short bowel syndrome. Symptoms include severe malnutrition and metabolic problems leading to weight loss, diarrhea, muscle wasting, dehydration, and electrolyte imbalances. The severity of the syndrome depends on how much and which sections of bowel are removed. Loss of the ileum is not tolerated as well as loss of the jejunum because of ileum's role in absorbing vitamin B-12. Other problems accompanying this syndrome can include excessive gastric acid due to loss of the buffering effects of the small intestine; increase in peristalsis due to loss of small intestine hormones that regulate bowel activity; formation of kidney stones due to excess oxalate absorption; and gallstone formation due to decrease in bile production.

Following resection, the remaining bowel has the ability to adapt to make up for loss of function. If adequate nutrition is provided for several months following surgery the bowel will gradually increase its absorptive surface area by forming larger villi and deeper crypts of Lieberkuhn. In the first several weeks after surgery, nutrition needs to be provided directly into the circulatory system of the patient. Gradually the patient may begin to receive nutritional support delivered into the stomach, duodenum, or jejunum. An easily digested liquid diet may be prescribed at first, avoiding sucrose and lactose. Vitamin supplementation with the fat-soluble vitamins is usually necessary, and vitamin B-12 status may need to be assessed depending on the area of resection. Supplementation with calcium, iron, and zinc may also be necessary. Several months after surgery oral intake may begin as tolerated. Setbacks are common and small meals are better tolerated than three main meals.

THE LIVER

LIVER CIRRHOSIS

Cirrhosis is the final stage of liver damage that occurs when normal liver tissue is gradually destroyed and replaced by scar tissue. This condition is found in 15% or more of heavy drinkers, but other causes may include poisoning, hepatitis, cystic fibrosis, or biliary obstruction. When normal tissue in the liver is replaced with connective or scar tissue, the liver becomes segmented with fibrous bands. Abnormal nodules form which limit blood circulation, and the damage is irreversible. Obstruction of the portal vein can cause pressure, which stimulates a new circulatory system to form that bypasses the damaged liver tissue. A consequence of this is the accumulation of fluid in the peritoneal cavity and enlargement of the veins providing the additional circulation. The pressure on these additional veins causes them to be thin-walled and places an individual at high risk of hemorrhage from venous rupture. Altered mental status can also occur due to toxins being carried across an abnormally porous blood-brain barrier.

In the case of light drinkers, alcohol can function as an additional energy source, providing 7 kcal/g, although no protein, fat, vitamins, or minerals are provided. In heavy drinkers, consumption of alcohol may take the place of food altogether. When alcohol is metabolized in the liver, triglycerides are formed which are deposited in the liver. Pyruvate metabolism is disrupted, and if glycogen stores are not being replenished the alcoholic may become hypoglycemic. Alcohol consumption causes inflammation of the stomach, pancreas, and intestine, which decreases the ability of these organs to absorb vitamin C, vitamin B-12, thiamin, and folic acid. Alcohol related thiamin deficiency is a common cause of dementia. When alcohol is metabolized to acetaldehyde, hepatic toxicity occurs, impairing the liver's ability to help the body use vitamins A, D, B-6, and folic acid. The problem in vitamin B impairment is furthered by the alcoholic's need for increased levels of the vitamin in the metabolism of alcohol.

NUTRITIONAL MANAGEMENT

Liver failure is defined as the function of the liver being reduced to 30% or less. The liver will no longer be able to absorb or metabolize fat properly, and the liver may become fatty. Fat should be reduced to 25% of caloric intake, and medium-chain triglycerides may be substituted for the more difficult-to-digest long chain fats. If medium-chain fats are used exclusively, supplementation with linoleic acid will avoid the development of an essential fatty acid deficiency. Fat in the stools is present in many cirrhotic patients due to lack of bile salts, pancreatic insufficiency, or portal vein blockage. This indicates the need for supplementation of the fat-soluble vitamins A, D, and E. In patients with advanced cirrhosis injections of vitamins A, D, and K may be necessary. Folate, thiamin, and vitamin-B12 deficiencies should also be addressed with supplementation. Due to liver impairment nutrient toxicities occur at low levels of supplementation so close monitoring is essential. Protein metabolism is greatly altered in advanced liver disease, and the ratio of aromatic amino acids to branched-chain amino acids (BCAA) becomes unbalanced, putting patients at risk for hepatic encephalopathy. However, this is complicated by the body's need for adequate protein to nourish the patient and provide building blocks for liver repair. Blood ammonia may be reduced by supplementing with neomycin, an antibiotic that destroys the flora in the gut that produces ammonia. Lactulose is also given, which removes intestinal contents by osmotically inducing diarrhea to help remove nitrogen. When these methods are unsuccessful supplementing protein intake with BCAA may help to improve encephalopathy. Ascites, or accumulation of fluid in the peritoneal cavity, can be managed by restricting sodium to 500-2000 mg/day, depending on the severity of the problem. Diuretics may also be given, and monitoring should include daily weight and abdominal examinations. As ascites dry up, normal fluid and sodium intake should resume.

GALLBLADDER

After bile is secreted by the liver, the gallbladder concentrates and stores the bile. The mucosa of the gallbladder absorbs water and electrolytes from the bile, leaving a concentrated product containing high levels of bile salts and cholesterol. Bile helps in the absorption of fats, vitamins A, D, E, and K, as well as calcium and iron. When food is ingested, the sphincter of Oddi relaxes, releasing bile into the duodenum through the common bile duct. The bile duct is joined with the liver and pancreatic ducts, so diseases involving the gallbladder often involve these other organs as well. The most common diseases of the gallbladder include gallstones (cholelithiasis) and inflammation (cholecystitis). Gallstones result from stones slipping into the common bile duct, causing cramps and pain. Inflammation can occur when gallstones block the duct opening, causing bile to back up into the gallbladder. The organ then becomes red, swollen, or possibly infected.

Surgery is usually the best treatment modality for gallbladder disease. The gallbladder is removed, and bile is stored in the common duct connecting the liver and small intestine. The duct expands to accommodate its new role, and bile moves directly from the liver to the small intestine. After surgery, enteral feedings may be offered until normal bowel sounds return, usually within the first few days. A low-fat diet may be followed for the first month after surgery, and then normal dietary intake may gradually resume as inflammation subsides.

Some patients are not surgical candidates, and must be treated conservatively with diet changes. For acute attacks of cholecystitis, the gallbladder should be rested by following a low-fat diet, as fat can painfully stimulate the sphincter of Oddi. For chronic disease, a diet providing 25% of kcal from fat may be followed, with supplementation of fat-soluble vitamins necessary in some individuals.

PANCREAS

The pancreas has cells that fall into the endocrine or exocrine category of functioning. The endocrine pancreas produces insulin, and the exocrine pancreas manufactures enzymes that help to digest carbohydrates, fats, and proteins in the intestine. Pancreatitis is an inflammation of the pancreas characterized by accumulation of pus in the intracellular space, fat necrosis, and edema. Pancreatitis can be acute or chronic, mild or severe enough to cause total loss of function. Symptoms can range from mild stomach discomfort to severe abdominal pain, shock, or even death. Diagnostic tests that may assess pancreatic function include checking for increased serum amylase levels, secretin stimulation test, 72-hour stool fat test, and glucose tolerance test. The exact cause is unknown but a leading contributing factor is alcoholism. The flow of pancreatic juice can be blocked, causing digestive juices to begin digesting the pancreas itself. Enzymes can also leak from the pancreas and begin to digest surrounding tissues.

NUTRITIONAL MANAGEMENT

The painful symptoms of pancreatitis flare up when pancreatic enzymes and bile are stimulated by the ingestion of food. When an individual is suffering from acute, severe pancreatitis all oral nutrition should cease and hydration should be given intravenously. 48 hours after the absence of severe symptoms clear liquids may be introduced slowly as tolerated. If the patient is unable to tolerate even a prescribed liquid diet containing a small amount of fat, glucose, and amino acids, parenteral nutrition is needed. In moderate attacks, several small meals a day with a very low-fat content may be offered. Chronic pancreatitis is characterized by failure of inflammation to subside or recurrent attacks. Large meals, high fat foods, and alcohol should be avoided. Over a period of several years, the function of the pancreas may deteriorate to the point that enzyme replacement is necessary. The enzyme pancrease can be given after meals to decrease the presence of fat in the stools.

Cystic Fibrosis

Cystic fibrosis is an inherited disease that involves a malfunction of the exocrine glands. This results in the production of thick, mucous-like secretions that obstruct the airway, pancreatic ducts, and ducts in other organs. Thick plugs block the pancreas from releasing digestive enzymes into the small intestine. This results in a cascade of negative effects, beginning with the malabsorption of all of the major nutrients. The excess mucous functions to further interfere with absorption. Damage to the pancreas over time can lead to diabetes. Patients may have poor oral intake due to shortness of breath and coughing, pain, weight loss accompanying infections, and impaired sense of smell. Enzyme replacement therapy is offered to control nutrient malabsorption. Calorie requirements are 120 to 150% of the RDA. High calorie snacks and larger portions at mealtimes should be offered. Fat malabsorption may require supplementation of fat-soluble vitamins. Sodium intake should be liberal to compensate for excess amounts lost in sweat.

Congestive Heart Failure

Congestive heart failure is the result of a long process of deterioration in which the heart loses its ability to function normally. The organ may be able to function in the early stages of disease by enlarging and increasing pulse rate. When normal blood circulation can no longer be maintained, patients experience shortness of breath, chest pain, and changes in blood pressure causing increased resorption of sodium and edema in the legs. Decreased blood flow to the brain can also cause altered mental status, headache, and anxiety.

Edema can disguise the disease in assessment by making typical anthropometric measures inaccurate. Dietary history and mid-upper arm circumference are appropriate tools. CHF patients experience decreased circulation to the kidneys, which allows sodium and fluid to accumulate in tissues. A low sodium diet and diuretics are needed to prevent further heart damage and to relieve edema. Use of diuretics can deplete potassium. Potassium supplementation may prevent digitalis toxicity.

Gestational Diabetes

Diabetes places additional stress on the body of the pregnant mother, and patients who previously controlled their glucose levels with diet alone may be required to take insulin. The goal is to meet the nutritional needs of the fetus, avoid large fluctuations of blood glucose during the day, and provide appropriate nutrition so that the mother's stores do not become exhausted. Babies born to diabetic women are larger, because the elevated glucose levels cross the placenta and result in overfeeding of the fetus. This results in increased insulin levels in the fetus, which can cause the newborn to become hypoglycemic after birth. In healthy women with normal pregnancies, the increased hormones secreted by the placenta stimulate the mother's body to produce more insulin. If the mother's body does not respond by secreting more insulin, gestational diabetes can result. All pregnant women should be screened using fasting glucose at 24 weeks gestation, and dietary management is usually effective.

Gout

Gout is a disease in which abnormal metabolism of purines result in excessive levels of uric acid in the blood. This results in the formation of sodium urate crystals, which accumulate in joints and cartilage. Over time, the excessive crystals can increase one's risk of kidney stones or cause damage in the joints, leading to arthritis. Obesity is a risk factor for developing gout, which is usually diagnosed after age 35. Both excessive eating and fasting resulting in ketosis can trigger attacks. Low purine diets are not effective in treating gout, as uric acid formation can occur within the body in the absence of purines. However, a low purine diet may be useful in acute attacks to reduce their severity. A gradual reduction in weight to ideal levels is recommended. A diet low in fat and

41

moderate in protein from sources low in purines like dairy and bread is recommended. Liberal intake of water is encouraged to dilute the uric acid in the urine.

GOITERS

If the thyroid gland does not produce enough T3 or T4 hormone, the pituitary gland may release additional thyroid stimulating hormone to try to up the thyroid's production. This causes an enlargement of the thyroid gland, or compensatory goiter. Endemic goiter is common in regions where iodine is absent from the diet. Iodine is stored in the thyroid where it is used to make T3 and T4 hormones. Iodine content is variable in foods; common sources include seafood, eggs, and milk. In areas where goiter is common, preparation of foods with iodized salt should be emphasized in order to reach the RDA of 150 micrograms/day. Goitrogens, substances in foods that block the absorption or use of iodine in the body, can also contribute to goiter. Goitrogen-rich foods include turnips, peanuts, and soybeans.

EPILEPSY

Epilepsy is a neurological disorder in which the cerebral neurons release excessive, disordered electrical discharges, causing a condition of chronic seizures. The anticonvulsant drugs Phenobarbital, phenytoin, and primidone increase the metabolism of vitamin D and therefore decrease the absorption of calcium in the intestine. Patients on these drugs are at an increased risk of osteomalacia and rickets, so vitamin D supplementation is necessary. Phenobarbital is absorbed poorly with meals, so the medication should be taken between meals.

A ketogenic diet is recommended as a last resort in some patients with moderate to severe seizures that cannot be adequately controlled by medication. The mechanism of action is thought to be an inhibitory effect of ketone bodies on neurotransmitters. The efficacy of the diet wears off after a few years. Nearly all of the energy needs in this diet are supplied by fat, and vitamin supplementation is required. The diet is unpalatable and side effects can include nausea and irritability, making compliance low.

FOOD ALLERGIES

IMMUNOLOGIC REACTION AND FOOD ALLERGIES

Usually, the gastrointestinal system and the immune system provide a barrier to proteins that have the ability to interact with the immune system and cause an allergic response. Foreign substances, or antigens, are cleared from the body by the immune system's macrophages, T lymphocytes, and B lymphocytes. The B lymphocytes play an important role in food allergies. These cells produce antibodies specific to antigens encountered in the body. Five types of antibodies are recognized: IgG, IgM, IgD, IgA, and IgE. When IgE antibodies bind with the allergen in special cells in the intestine, skin, and respiratory tract, chemicals are released that begin what is recognized as an allergic reaction. Histamine, bradykinin, and serotonin can cause abdominal pain, coughing, or itching in mild reactions; anaphylaxis, shock, and death can occur in severe cases. The symptoms can begin within seconds of ingesting the offending food or up to two hours later. Common culprits include eggs, fish, wheat, soy, peanuts, and milk.

DIAGNOSTIC PROCEDURES

There is no catchall test used to diagnose food allergies, so several tests are usually done to pinpoint the offender. A diet history is taken to determine the symptoms, a list of foods that were ingested around symptom development, duration between consumption and symptom development, and family history of allergies. A two-week food and symptom diary provided by the patient is helpful. The *skin prick test* is a reliable immunologic test that cannot be used alone, but can help narrow down suspicious foods to use in a food challenge. A welt larger than 3mm from a skin test is useful for children over three years of age; younger children may not have positive skin test reactions to allergens. A *double-blind food challenge* can help to identify multiple food allergies. The food is administered in capsule form, along with a placebo, and neither the patient nor the health professional knows which capsule has been offered until the end of the test.

BURNS

Extensive burns can increase basal energy expenditure by 100% or more. Protein catabolism and nitrogen excretion are increased, and protein is also lost through the wound itself. Fluid and electrolyte losses from the wound can be severe, and the initial treatment period should focus on replacing fluid and electrolytes and maintaining balance. Calculation of kcal requirements can be determined by various formulas that consider kcal/kg and total body surface area burned. Additional energy is required to meet the demands of wound healing, fever, infection, weight loss, and surgery. Protein needs are increased and may be determined by monitoring the patient's wound status and nitrogen balance. Vitamin C supplementation is helpful for the collagen formation needed in wound healing. Magnesium can be lost from wounds in large levels; supplementation may be necessary. Zinc is recommended for those receiving parenteral nutrition or for those with deficiencies to enhance wound healing.

INJURY RECOVERY

Nutritional support for accident victims should begin as soon as the patient's vital signs are stable. Although positive nitrogen balance may not be achieved in the first days following trauma, further loss of lean body tissue may be prevented. Introduction of oral feeding may be delayed due to shock, pain, injury complications, or depression. Enteral nutrition is routinely given to avoid complications of protein loss that include hypoalbuminemia, infection, slow wound healing, skin breakdown, and reduced immune function. The degree of trauma determines the amount of carbohydrate and protein needed. Most patients' needs are satisfied by 35-45 kcal/kg. Lipid should provide ~30% of kcal, and protein needs vary from 1-2 g/kg, depending on severity of injury.

Individuals recovering from surgery generally delay oral feeding for 24-48 hours, to wait for normal peristalsis to return. Fluid and electrolyte balance should be monitored postoperatively and maintained intravenously as needed. Positive nitrogen balance enhances wound healing and reduces infection; most patients can meet their energy and protein needs on the standard diet provided.

OBESITY

The body mass index ($BMI=W/H^2$, weight in kg and height in m) is the preferred measure for determining whether an individual is overweight or obese. A BMI of 30 or greater classifies an individual as obese. A BMI of 25-29.9 classifies one as overweight. A variety of factors may contribute to the condition of obesity, including environment, culture, heredity, and internal physiological differences. Many variables that determine the individual regulation of body weight are genetically determined, such as resting metabolic rate, amount and size of fat cells, and subtle hormonal and neurological factors that control the feeling of satiety. The set point theory argues that people have a predetermined weight, which is governed by fat stores in the body, and individuals will achieve homeostasis by returning to this weight over time regardless of feeding habits. Obesity is associated with a range of diseases and disorders, including hypertension, diabetes, heart disease, gallstones, and arthritis.

NUTRITIONAL CARE

Treatment of overweight patients may be viewed as caring for a chronic disease, as few individuals maintain their weight. Weight cycling refers to the trait of obese persons to lose weight and regain it several times over their life. Typically, more weight is regained than was lost, and the composition of weight regained tends to be higher in adipose tissue and lower in lean muscle mass. Successful weight loss programs usually integrate diet, exercise, and behavior change. Many dieting individuals experience a "plateau effect," where weight reduction slows or stops completely. Loss of muscle used to support fatty tissue contributes to a reduction of resting metabolic rate. Steady weight loss over a long period of time helps to conserve lean body mass and reduce fat stores. Achievement of ideal body weight may not be possible for individuals with a BMI >40, so final goals should be individualized. A diet that provides 500 kcal/day less than required for maintenance should provide weight loss of ~1 lb. a week.

CHEMOTHERAPY

Chemotherapy is a systemic treatment, and side effects vary according to the drugs and dosage used. Chemotherapy kills rapidly dividing cells, so the entire GI tract may be affected, leading to nausea, vomiting, diarrhea, mouth sores, and inflammation of the esophagus. The patient can become severely anorectic due to taste aversions caused by metallic taste and nausea. Patients may associate eating with pain, nausea, and vomiting to such an extent that formerly favorite foods are rejected, and cooking odors alone can trigger GI upset. Food service workers may be instructed not to remove tray lids in the patient's room in the hospital setting, as the subsequent release of food odors leads to rejection. Meat aversion is especially common, so protein sources may need to come from bland dairy foods, like cottage cheese. Serving foods cold or at room temperature can increase their appeal. If malnutrition becomes severe or the gut loses function, temporary enteral or parenteral nutrition may be required.

DENTAL CARIES

Dental caries form when bacteria in the mouth ferment dietary carbohydrates, especially sucrose, causing the formation of acids. The acids decalcify the surface of the tooth until salivary flow clears food debris from the mouth and the buffering action provided by the lower pH of saliva neutralizes the acids. Saliva also contains calcium and phosphorus, which help to remineralize eroded areas after a meal. If the acid is trapped in plaque formations on the teeth, the acid production may continue for an hour after the meal. When pH drops below 5.5, the acid is able to destroy tooth enamel. The frequency of consumption of cariogenic food affects caries formation. Eating a large portion of dessert is less damaging than snacking throughout the day. Sticky foods that adhere to the tooth are more cariogenic. The amount of time the food is in the mouth provides opportunities for bacteria to act, so liquids are less cariogenic than solid foods. Cheddar cheese and sugarless gum have been shown to prevent the drop of pH in the mouth.

AIDS

AIDS is caused by the blood-borne virus HIV, which destroys T lymphocyte function and therefore causes severe immune deficiency. The virus is also transmitted through breast milk, so HIV positive mothers should not nurse. The disease is associated with susceptibility to various opportunistic infections, lymphoma, Kaposi's sarcoma, and encephalopathy. Organs affected by the complications of AIDS can include the liver, kidneys, GI tract, and pancreas. Oral candidiasis is common in AIDS patients, which makes eating painful. Energy needs are increased in patients with infections or febrile illness, yet oral intake can be poor due to nausea, vomiting, or fatigue. The protein malnutrition common to AIDS patients can further increase their susceptibility to infections. However, protein intake may be restricted for those with renal disease. Goals of nutritional care include preservation of protein stores, prevention of vitamin or mineral deficiencies that reduce immune status, and treatment of complications that compromise nutritional status.

COPD

Chronic obstructive pulmonary disease is the airway obstruction that develops as a result of chronic bronchitis and/or emphysema. Chronic bronchitis is characterized by a productive cough that may come and go but never resolves. Emphysema is a condition characterized by enlarged alveoli (air sacs) that exhibit degraded walls and a loss of elasticity. Patients with severe COPD are at risk for cor pulmonale, a condition in which the right ventricle of the heart is enlarged due to increased pressure in the pulmonary arteries. The malnourished state common to COPD patients is thought to be a result of increased energy needs, anorexia, and increased oxygen consumption. The goals of nutritional support include maintaining ideal body weight, managing medication side effects, and managing the edema of patients with cor pulmonale. Edema can mask weight loss, so assessment should account for this. Some edematous patients can achieve control with sodium and fluid restriction; others need diuretics. Energy requirements may approach 150% of resting energy expenditure. High-calorie liquid supplements may help patients reach their energy intake goals.

NUTRITION DIAGNOSTIC LABELING
LABELING

The clinical domain in the nutrition diagnostic labeling process: When conducting a nutrition diagnosis, the dietitian may identify nutritional problems in the patient that relate to the medical problem the patient is experiencing; this is not to be confused with a medical diagnosis. The clinical domain encompasses three classes: functional balance, biochemical balance, and weight balance:

- *Functional balance* problems can be physical or mechanical and interfere with one's ability to achieve normal nutritional status, for example, inability to chew.
- *Biochemical balance* represents a loss of the ability to metabolize foods normally, due to medicine, surgery, or a disease process. An example would be the malabsorption of short bowel syndrome.
- *Weight balance* describes involuntary weight changes that deviate from the patient's normal or desired body weight. This includes excessive weight loss or gain.

Components of the intake domain in nutrition diagnostic labeling: The intake domain of nutrition diagnosis includes problems related to the ingestion of energy, vitamins, minerals, and fluids, whether the patient receives nutrition orally, enterally, or parenterally. This domain encompasses five classes of concern:

- *Calorie energy balance* is used to describe observed or potential changes in energy expenditure, due to diagnoses such as anorexia, dialysis, trauma, or other conditions that can place one in catabolic or anabolic state.
- *Oral or nutrition support intake* is described as adequate or excessive compared to the goal.
- *Fluid intake balance* is also described as adequate or excessive compared to the goal. This can be significant in many disease processes of the kidney, where fluid intake is strictly regulated.
- *Bioactive substance charting* gives the dietitian an opportunity to chart miscellaneous substances ingested by the patient, such as vitamin supplements or alcohol.
- *Nutrient balance* expands on the patient's use of vitamin or mineral supplements by examining the practice of ingesting large amounts of single nutrients, as is sometimes done with vitamin C.

Behavioral-environmental domain in nutrition diagnostic labeling: The behavioral-environmental domain describes problems or findings that relate to a patient's knowledge, attitudes, beliefs, environment, food safety, or access to food. Knowledge and beliefs may encompass cultural practices that are harmful to one's nutritional status, such as the Native American's practice of feeding sugar-sweetened beverages in bottles to young children, leading to dental decay. Examples of concerns in the class of physical activity balance and function might include an elderly person no longer able to prepare food, or a sedentary person whose inactivity places him or her at risk for obesity. Food safety and access encompasses problems related to the ability to obtain the foods needed to maintain good nutrition and the ability to store and prepare food safely. A homeless person unable to refrigerate foods would be described in this category.

PESS STATEMENT

When charting a patient's nutrition diagnosis, the dietitian should describe the problem in standardized language that includes the problem, etiology, signs, and symptoms. In order to write the problem, a dietitian must use an approved diagnostic label. This is a statement that includes an adjective to capture how the patient deviates from the desired state of health. Examples include "altered mental status," "impaired bowel function," "chronic renal failure," or "at risk of liver cirrhosis." The next step is to define the etiology, or the cause/contributing risk factors that contribute to the problem. The appropriate way to chart this is to use the language "related to." Contributing factors in etiology may be physical, situational, cultural, developmental, or anything found to be an underlying cause of the problem. The last step is to chart the signs and symptoms present in the patient. This may include findings from lab tests, anthropometric measures, or descriptions given by the patient.

Planning and Intervention

INTERVENTIONS AND PREVENTIONS

Nutrition intervention and evidence-based dietetics practice:

Nutrition intervention encompasses those actions or steps a dietitian takes to change a behavior, counter a risk factor, or improve a condition he or she encounters in the individual or community being assessed.

Evidence-based dietetics practice is one of the tools used in nutrition care to prevent disease and enhance health in patients. This type of practice uses the ability to glean what is most important in the medical literature and combine that information with patient values and professional knowledge in order to provide effective treatment to individuals. The tool adds credibility to the profession of dietetics in that not only must the dietitian be able to find the best evidence to support his or her clinical decisions, the dietitian must also view the data through a critical lens in order to choose the best course of action.

SPECIFIC DIET TYPES

THERAPEUTIC

A therapeutic diet is one that is specifically designed to meet a patient's needs. Therapeutic diets vary widely and may include orders to increase consumption of certain nutrients to presentation/adaptation of regularly served menu items. Generally, the facility diet manual will guide the physician in preparing his/her dietary orders. Though other healthcare team members are often consulted in regards to a patient's needs, a therapeutic diet may only be ordered or changed by a physician. Once that diet is ordered, a nutrition specialist and/or dietary manager will generally oversee the manner in which the doctor's orders are implemented. Again, it is important to remember, that ONLY the physician may change, modify, or cancel a dietary order. Any questions regarding the order should be directed to the ordering physician and/or his staff dietitian.

HIGH CALORIE, HIGH PROTEIN

A high calorie, high protein diet is most often ordered for patients who have suffered a high degree of weight loss in a short period of time, those who were not able to eat anything by mouth over an extended period of time, and/or in failure to thrive cases. Physicians/nutritionists often recommend that cancer patients adhere to a high calorie, high protein diet in order to maintain their strength and combat fatigue during treatment. High calorie, high fat diets encourage consumption of whole dairy products, such as whole milk, ice cream, butter, and cream. Peanut butter, meats, nuts, avocado, and other similar foods may be great supplements to this diet.

LACTOSE INTOLERANCE

Lactose is the primary sugar found in milk products. An individual who exhibits lactose intolerance lacks the enzyme that breaks down the lactose to an easily digestible form. Individuals who are lactose intolerant should avoid many dairy products but should still strive to meet daily calcium recommendations. Calcium may be garnered through other sources, such as by consuming dark, green vegetables, soy, tofu, salmon, sardines, beans, and oranges. Some individuals are able to tolerate yogurt with live bacteria cultures as the bacteria has the enzyme necessary to breakdown the lactose.

**Note: Many non-dairy, processed foods may also contain lactose, which was added during the preparation process. Additionally, vitamins, supplements, and prescription drugs may also contain lactose.

VEGETARIAN

Vegetarians rely on plant sources as their primary source of food. There are three types of vegetarian diets. Those diets are as follows: *vegan* diets exclude all animal meats and products; *lacto-vegetarian* diets allow consumption of plant and dairy products; and the *lacto-ovo-vegetarian* diet incorporates dairy, egg, and plant products. Vegetarians often need to supplement their diet with alternative sources of calcium, protein, iron, and B12 vitamin. Tofu, soy, and nuts are helpful protein and calcium supplements. Enriched cereals and other grains are also helpful supplements to any of the above diets.

LOW CHOLESTEROL

Low cholesterol diets are often used to help combat cardiovascular disease by controlling or reducing blood lipid and cholesterol levels. Typically, low cholesterol diets aim to limit cholesterol intake to 200-300 milligrams per day. By limiting or eliminating high cholesterol foods, one can easily lower the risk of heart disease. Cholesterol is only found in animal products. That is to say, cholesterol may be found in meats, poultry, seafood, eggs, and dairy products. Conversely, cholesterol is not present in plant products, even those with high fat content. Organ meats, especially liver, and eggs have particularly high cholesterol contents. To implement a low cholesterol diet, a client may limit animal product consumption and/or eat lean cuts of meat and low-fat dairy products. Additionally, adding more fruits, vegetables, and whole grains to the diet will help lower cholesterol.

KOSHER

Practicing Orthodox Jews observe a kosher diet. That diet is derived from biblical texts in which certain foods are permitted and others are outlawed. Foods avoided by those on a kosher diet include meats such as pork and rabbit, seafood such as catfish, shellfish, and shrimp, certain types of foul, and any type of insect. Kosher regulations also include specific rules forbidding dairy products from coming in contact with meat, as well as specific regulations regarding cheese, wine, and some juices. Moreover, kosher foods must be prepared in a humane and painless manner, with a rabbi overseeing the animal slaughter. One should look for foods labeled kosher when preparing meals for a client on a kosher diet. Frequently, non-kosher foods are tainted by an ingredient derived from a non-kosher source.

ISLAMIC

Similar to Orthodox Jews, Muslims practice certain dietary restrictions and observe a diet called Halal. Halal diets are very similar to kosher diets. Foods that are forbidden include pork, carnivorous and omnivorous animals, certain fowl, non-amphibious animals without external ears, and blood products. Muslims are allowed to eat fish-eating animals. Additionally, all permissible animal products must be properly slaughtered under the auspices of an expert. Halal diets also forbid any consumption of alcohol. Again, as with kosher diets, Halal diets are often exclusionary of prepared foods as ingredient sources may be unknown and/or improperly prepared.

KETOGENIC DIET

The ketogenic diet gets its name because the high fat content of the diet results in conversion of fat-to-ketones that are utilized as an energy source in place of glucose. If carbohydrates (which are composed of sugars) are eliminated from the diet, and a diet very high in fat is substituted, the body has no dietary sources of glucose. As a result, ketones are made from the available sources and these are used as fuel instead. It is necessary to be scrupulous in the restriction of carbohydrates because even a very small amount of sugar can cause the body to shift to glucose production and use, which it prefers to ketones.

For example, this restriction is such that children on the diet have to be careful to take sugarless daily multivitamins. Supplements of folate, B_6, B_{12}, vitamin D, and Ca are required with this diet. The ketogenic diet is often used in the treatment of epilepsy or seizure disorders.

HEMODIALYSIS DIET

The hemodialysis diet is an eating plan tailored to patients who are in stage 5 of chronic kidney disease (CKD), also known as end-stage renal disease (ESRD). These patients have very little or no kidney function and must undergo dialysis to clean their blood of waste and excess fluids. Hemodialysis is one type of dialysis. The procedure is done several times a week, usually for 3 to 4 hours at a time. The hemodialysis diet is designed to reduce the amount of fluid and waste that builds up between hemodialysis treatments. The hemodialysis diet will restrict foods that contain high amounts of sodium, phosphorus, and potassium. The hemodialysis diet will introduce a higher amount of protein into the eating plan. Certain fruits, vegetables, dairy products, and other foods that are very high in potassium will need to be restricted on the hemodialysis diet. Recommended 1.2 g protein/kg.

PERITONEAL DIALYSIS DIET

The peritoneal dialysis (PD) diet is designed for patients who choose PD instead of hemodialysis. It is a slightly different diet than the hemodialysis diet, because of the differences in the dialysis treatments. Unlike hemodialysis, PD is performed daily. As a result, the body does not buildup as much potassium, sodium, and fluid, so the diet is more liberal. Protein requirements are higher, because protein is lost through the peritoneal membrane. Patients on PD are at risk for infection, so a diet with adequate protein is needed to keep the body strong. Unlike hemodialysis patients, PD patients are likely to keep normal or low potassium levels. Patients may be encouraged to eat potassium-rich foods such as tomatoes, orange juice, and bananas if their blood test levels are too low. The peritoneal dialysis diet is not as restricted in sodium and fluid compared with the diet for hemodialysis, because dialysis is performed daily. Recommend 1.2 to 1.3 g protein/kg.

HYPERTENSION

Hypertension is defined as a systolic blood pressure of 140 or greater and a diastolic blood pressure of 90 or greater. Blood pressure levels are managed in the body by a variety of mechanisms, including the volume of fluid in the vascular system, the contractions of the heart pushing the blood through the blood vessels, and the strength of the muscular walls of the arterioles. Several organs work in coordination to maintain normal blood pressure levels, including the kidney, heart, and nervous system.

If the kidney is unable to excrete excess sodium, the elevated sodium and water levels in the blood cause an increased plasma volume. The increase in sodium in cells may also cause a rise in calcium in the vessel musculature, increasing rigidity and raising pressure. Obese persons have a higher risk for hypertension, perhaps due to the increased insulin levels triggering the kidneys to increase sodium reabsorption.

MANAGING HYPERTENSION THROUGH MEDICATION AND DIET

The standard pharmacological approach for the management of hypertension is the administration of diuretics and antihypertensive drugs. Diuretics can lower the volume of fluid in the circulation and decrease sodium in the body. However, potassium loss can be an unwanted effect of treatment with thiazide diuretics, increasing the possibility of hypokalemia. Additional potassium should be given unless potassium-sparing drugs are used. Conservative treatment for mild cases of hypertension includes using weight loss, low sodium diet, alcohol reduction, and aerobic exercise. Even moderate weight loss can reduce the activity of the sympathetic nervous system, which plays a big role in blood pressure management. Reducing sodium intake to less than 1500mg/day or less can help the individuals who are truly salt sensitive; in others it may help the medications work more effectively. The consumption of three or more drinks a day is the cause of a small percentage of reversible hypertension, especially in women, so moderation in intake is appropriate.

METABOLIC DISORDERS

Galactosemia is a metabolic disorder that describes two different syndromes that make the body unable to convert galactose into glucose. This causes the accumulation of galactose and/or galactose-1 phosphate in body tissues or intercellular fluid. Galactosemia occurs when one of two enzyme activities that ultimately allow lactose to be broken down into glucose is not functioning. If the galactose-1-phosphate uridyl transferase enzyme is dysfunctional at birth, infants may present with vomiting, diarrhea, susceptibility to infections, and failure to thrive. If not diagnosed and treated promptly death can occur. Nutritional management includes lifelong galactose elimination from the diet. This includes avoiding all dairy products, dates, bell peppers, organ meats, and papaya.

Urea cycle defects, including OTC deficiency, citrullinemia, and Argininosuccinic aciduria result in accumulations of ammonia in the blood that can cause vomiting, seizures, and death. The goal of therapy is to prevent excessive ammonia in the blood and accompanying neurological deficits. Acute attacks may require the elimination of all dietary protein, while long-term management restricts protein from 1-2 g/day.

ACUTE RESPIRATORY DISTRESS SYNDROME

Acute respiratory failure can occur in patients with chronic obstructive pulmonary disease when the respiratory muscle is no longer strong enough to enable the lungs to exchange enough gases to keep blood oxygen at functioning levels. Patients with this condition usually have poor nutritional status and are at risk for worsening their status during hospitalization. Patients who can improve their protein levels have a better chance of weaning from mechanical ventilation. Goals include preserving lean body mass, preventing further weight loss, and maintaining fluid balance, while taking into account the patient's impaired ability to clear carbon dioxide from the body. Increased carbohydrate in the diet is associated with increased carbon dioxide production, so 50% of the non-protein calories provided should come from fat. Enteral feedings are recommended for patients with a functional gut, but care in tube placement should be taken to avoid the risk of aspiration.

ENTERAL FEEDING

Enteral feeding is any method of tube feeding where food is delivered directly to the stomach. There are several different types of tubes, and the type of tube may dictate the location of the device. For example, the tube may be inserted in various positions of the stomach or along other areas of the gastro-intestinal tract. Enteral tubes increase the risk of infection in patients, as there is essentially an open line between one's environment and stomach. Therefore, feeding assistants should use the utmost care, to include hand washing and sanitization, utilizing sanitized equipment, properly flushing and caring for the tube, and following any procedures specific to the patient, when assisting with tube feedings. Enteral tubes are most often used in patients who have lost their ability to swallow and/or have diminished peristalsis.

ENTERAL FEEDING FORMULAS

Enteral feeding may be the choice for those unable to maintain nutrition orally due to surgery, dysphagia, coma, or esophageal obstruction. The GI tract must still be functional, with >2 feet of working small intestine. Formulas may be commercially prepared, which offers convenience, consistency, and reduced expense, but individually prepared solutions may better meet the needs of some patients. Modular formulas are composed from varying amounts of carbohydrate, fat, protein, vitamins, minerals, and water. Enteral feedings can also be made from whole foods that have been pureed and strained. Advantages of this method include reduced cost and presence of trace nutrients; disadvantages include increased chance of contamination and the need for a larger feeding tube. Patients with malabsorption from short-bowel syndrome or other diseases may need defined formulas, which are easier to digest due to the simpler energy forms they contain. Glucose or dextrins provide carbohydrates, amino acids provide protein, and monoglycerides and diglycerides provide lipids. Most enteral formulas provide 1-1.5 kcal/cc.

POSSIBLE COMPLICATIONS

If a patient has more than three episodes of diarrhea a day, several feeding-related problems may be at fault. Patients should be assessed for lactose intolerance, and offered lactose-free formula if needed. Formula should be discarded every 24 hours to avoid diarrhea from bacterial contamination. If formula has high osmolarity or is being infused too rapidly, continuous drip may be appropriate. If nausea or vomiting occurs, this may indicate that the GI tract is not functioning. Repositioning the tube into the duodenum may help, or parenteral feeding may be necessary. If patient is aspirating the formula after feeding, there is a risk of pneumonia. This may be prevented by elevating the patient's head during feeding, changing to a lower bore (smaller) tube, or placing the tube in the duodenum. Obstruction of the feeding tube may be suspected if the patient does not receive more than 12 hours of a feeding. Frequent flushing of the tube or changing to a large bore tube can help prevent this.

PARENTERAL FEEDING

Parenteral feeding is a method of feeding in which nutrients are delivered directly to the blood stream through the use of a catheter. Parenteral feeding completely bypasses the digestive system and is frequently used in patients who have had part of their digestive system removed or are having severe problems digesting foods and are lacking essential nutrients. Like patients who receive enteral feedings, those receiving parenteral feedings are highly susceptible to infection, and therefore, feedings must be handled with the utmost of care by the patient and caregivers. Additionally, the patient's environment should be kept extremely clean. The nutrients delivered parenterally are combined to create a specific formula. Various drugs may affect the formulas and should be carefully added to patient's regimen.

PARENTERAL FORMULAS

For protein synthesis and anabolism to take place, the TPN solution can provide 1 gram of protein for every 150 calories. For severely stressed patients, the solution may be adjusted to provide 1 gram of protein/100 calories. Protein is provided by crystalline amino acids. Common solutions range from 5-15% amino acids. The types of amino acids can be adjusted according to the disease state. For example, branched-chain amino acids can be used in solutions for patients with liver failure, and essential amino acid-rich formulas are given to patients with kidney failure. Carbohydrate is usually provided in the form of dextrose, which has a higher osmolality than glucose. No more than 4 or 5 mg/kg/minute should be given to prevent hyperglycemia and excessive carbon dioxide production. Lipids provide 25-35% of calories to avoid essential fatty acid deficiency. Potassium may be increased in high anabolic states to balance the movement of potassium into the cells. Phosphorus is important when high calorie solutions are given to prevent hypophosphatemia.

TRANSITIONAL FEEDING

Transitional feeding refers to the period when a patient switches from parenteral to enteral or oral feeding, or from enteral to oral feeding. Patients are at risk for hypophosphatemia during this time, and must be monitored closely. When patients have been without food for a period of time, aggressive refeeding causes phosphorus to rapidly leave the plasma and enter the cell in order to take part in the manufacture of adenosine triphosphate. The risk is increased in alcoholics, diabetics, and patients with kidney disease. Phosphate supplementation may be necessary to prevent severe metabolic and hematological side effects. Patients may also experience low levels of potassium as cellular needs increase, so monitoring and supplementation as necessary should occur. Intestinal enzyme counts are low after a period of no food, and patients may not tolerate lactose at first. First meals should be lactose-free, low in sodium and carbohydrate, and supplemented with electrolytes as needed.

LONG-TERM CARE

In a long-term care setting, a care plan is developed after the initial assessment. The initial assessment must be completed within fourteen days of patient admittance. Then, the care plan is developed to ensure that the client's needs are met. This care plan includes any special dietary orders, including prescription of a therapeutic diet, and it must be completed within seven days of the completion of the initial assessment. Thus, within 21 days of admittance to a long-term care facility, every patient should have a personalized care plan. Assuming that there are no changes in a patient's health, the care plan must be updated quarterly. Otherwise, the care plan should be revisited with every significant change in the patient's health.

CHOLESTEROL MANAGEMENT

The Adult Treatment Panel (ATP) III is the National Cholesterol Education Program's clinical guidelines for cholesterol testing and management. The program periodically updates its ATP reports based on advances in cholesterol research, and the third report focuses on prevention of coronary heart disease in people with multiple risk factors.

This report informs health practitioners that elevated LDL cholesterol levels are the main contributing cause to heart disease. The first step in prevention is determining the individual's risk, with a complete lipoprotein profile for all adults older than 20 years of age being recommended. LDL cholesterol levels below 100 are optimal. Smokers, hypertensive people, diabetics, and those with a family history of CHD have the highest risk and should strive for optimal levels. The program recommends reducing saturated fat and cholesterol intake, exercise, and weight control. The therapeutic lifestyle diet (TLC) calls for increased fiber intake (10 to 25 g/day), lowered saturated fat intake (less than 7% calories), and lowered cholesterol intake (less than 200 mg/day). Moderate physical activity and maintaining normal body weight are also advocated.

ADA NUTRITION CARE PROCESS

The NCP is designed to meet changing nutritional needs. The process may be initiated by the referral of a doctor who discovers a patient experiencing or at risk for nutrition-related problems. The methods used in this type of care require the use of critical thinking and problem-solving skills. The process is made up of assessment of nutritional status, diagnosis of nutritional needs or problems, implementation of interventions necessary to meet care objectives, and monitoring and evaluation of the nutritional care. The rationale of the NCP is to give dietitians a common structure and method to promote better decision making and to obtain data that may be evaluated quantitatively and qualitatively. The process also serves to validate the care provided by dietitians and allows for continual improvement in the nutrition care cycle.

Dietitians should think about verbal or nonverbal cues the patient provides so that they can tailor their interview appropriately. When thinking about which data to collect and which tools to use, the information gathered should be accurate, appropriate to the patient, and interpreted using only those tools and methods pertinent to the situation. Types of data collected should be relevant to the situation and may cover such broad concerns as health, nutritional, functional, and behavioral status. Documentation should be organized and should exclude information that does not help to identify nutrition-related problems or concerns. The screening and assessment should also help the dietitian identify when consultation with other health professionals is needed. The NCP process does not end with the initial screening but is an ongoing process that may require repeated assessments until a reason for discharge or discontinuation of therapy is reached.

SOP, SOPP, AND SODPF

The Standards of Practice in Nutrition Care (SOP), Standards of Professional Performance (SOPP), and the Scope of Dietetic Practice Framework (SODPF) all work together to support quality dietetic practice according to the philosophy set forth by the Nutrition Care Process and Model. The SODPF is not a list of services that one is or is not authorized to perform; rather, it is a dynamic framework that encompasses the knowledge base, ethics, research, education, and standards of care that make up the profession of dietetics. SOP includes the range of services that a dietitian might provide in a safe, sanctioned setting. SOPP describes the satisfactory behavior one should execute when acting in the professional role of dietitian. It can be used within the profession to evaluate one's own performance, by administrators to determine if patient needs are being met, or by human resources departments to make hiring and employment decisions.

HEALTHY PEOPLE 2030 PROGRAM

Healthy People 2030 is a set of goals and objectives set forth by the Surgeon General to encourage the health of the nation by focusing on disease prevention. Local and regional governments can use these objectives to develop programs that encourage behavior change for the sake of improving health. The main goals of the program are to improve the quality and length of life, and to eliminate health disparities among different populations. The program encompasses 62 focal areas, ranging from food safety to chronic kidney disease to maternal, infant, and child health. These focal areas are grouped into five main topic areas: health conditions, health behaviors, populations, settings and systems, and social determinants of health. The focal areas allow organizations to choose the focus area that pertains to their population in developing interventions and programs. Particular indicators within a focus area are selected to serve as progress markers, and objective measures allow educators, policy makers, and researchers to assess how well the goals are being met. For example, in the overweight and obesity category, one goal recommends that children receive 60 minutes or more of physical activity per day.

USDA PROGRAMS

COMMODITY FOOD DONATION/DISTRIBUTION PROGRAM

The USDA's Commodity Food Programs serve the dual function of providing food to individuals who need it, and to help American farmers by providing a market for their goods. The Commodity Supplemental Food Program provides nutrition for those deemed to be at highest risk: low-income women, children under the age of six, and the elderly. Qualifying individuals receive a monthly package containing such items as canned meats and vegetables, cereal, and juice. This is not meant to provide for all of their nutritional needs, but may help those on the edge of food insecurity.

The Emergency Food Assistance Program distributes foods purchased by the USDA to each state, where it is then distributed to local food banks. Foods are then distributed to soup kitchens or directly to households. The amount received by each state depends on the number of unemployed and low-income citizens in that state. This program is meant to serve as a temporary emergency aid to recipients, not a permanent solution.

NATIONAL SCHOOL LUNCH PROGRAM

Established by President Truman in 1946, the National School Lunch Program works to ensure the health of the nation's children by providing free or reduced cost lunches to public schools, nonprofit private schools, and residential child care facilities. Qualifying schools receive federal subsidies in turn for providing nutritionally balanced meals to students who meet income guidelines. Children from families with incomes between 130% and 185% of the poverty level receive lunches for free or reduced prices, and non-qualifying children must pay full price, although the programs must not operate for profit. The foodservice program decides what food is served, but lunches must provide 1/3 of the nutrients specified by the Dietary Guidelines for Americans. Schools get additional support in the form of commodity foods available from local surplus stock. Team Nutrition USDA further supports schools by providing nutrition training, recipes and menus, and other educational assistance.

SCHOOL BREAKFAST PROGRAM, SPECIAL MILK PROGRAM, AND SUMMER FOOD PROGRAM

The USDA's Food and Nutrition Service has been in operation since 1975, providing cash reimbursement to schools that provide free or low-cost breakfasts to qualifying low-income students. The meal provides ¼ of the daily requirements for nutrients, and the USDA's Team Nutrition helps the food service staff of schools with menu planning and other training and educational efforts.

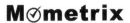

The USDA's Special Milk Program provides milk to children who do not participate in other federal meal programs. The program is meant to encourage consumption of milk among children, and schools are reimbursed for the milk they provide. The program also contributes to the nourishment of children who attend abbreviated schedule classes where meal programs are not available. The USDA's Summer Food Program helps fill the gap when school ends for summer break. This program combines wholesome meals with summer activities in sites like camps or community centers. Children may receive up to three meals a day if enrolled in residential camps.

CHILD AND ADULT CARE FOOD PROGRAM (CACFP)

CACFP provides meals and snacks to low-income children and impaired elderly individuals enrolled in daycare settings. The program also provides snacks to low-income children enrolled in after-school care. Those in daycare may receive up to two meals and one snack; after-school participants under age 18 can receive one snack per day. An exception is homeless shelters, which can provide three meals a day to children residing there. The program covers both public and private care settings, including personal residents providing in-home daycare. Reimbursement varies, and may be calculated as a percentage, per meal count, or blended per meal rates. Additional funds are provided to centers to cover costs incurred in the planning and implementing of the program. The USDA provides recipes and purchased commodities to assist those after-school care facilities with limited food preparation areas.

WIC PROGRAM

The Special Supplemental Nutrition Program for Women, Infants, and Children (WIC) provides nutritious foods, nutrition counseling, and referrals to other social service agencies for services like immunizations for woman and children. Services are provided in all 50 states through sites such as community centers, health departments, schools, hospitals, and mobile clinics. Funds are not available for every possible eligible person to participate, and eligibility is determined by income, level of nutritional risk, and whether the person fits into the categories of individuals served. Pregnant women and women 6-12 months postpartum are served, depending on breastfeeding status. Infants up to age of one year are a focus of the program, but children up to age five may qualify. Participants may be deemed to be at nutritional risk after a health screening identifies such problems as anemia, weight problems, or a history of pregnancy complications. Food packages provided through the program contain such items as cow's milk, 100% juice, infant formula, and iron-fortified cereal.

HEALTHY START AND HEAD START

Healthy Start was initiated in 1991 with the goal of improving the health of pregnant women and reducing infant mortality for populations affected by a higher than average infant mortality rate. Clinics provide free prenatal care to women within their community, using mobile clinics when necessary. The period between pregnancies is targeted as an ideal time when women can be counseled or treated for problems that may affect future pregnancies, such as substance abuse, obesity, or diabetes.

Head Start is a program for children birth through age five, with a focus on preschool aged children that prepares them for school by providing them with nutritional, health, social, and educational services. Parents are not served directly but are encouraged to get involved in their children's learning process. Nutritionists involved in head start monitor food-related activities within the program, teach the parents how to prepare healthy foods at home, and instill an appreciation for healthy foods in the children.

FOOD STAMP PROGRAM

The Food Stamp Program provides qualifying individuals with coupons or a debit-like card that can be used like cash at the grocery store to increase the buying power of needy families. Reimbursements are determined in part based on the USDA's Thrifty Food Plan, which reflects foods that will meet dietary recommendations at the lowest cost. The program is administered by state and local agencies, although the federal government covers the majority of the cost. Eligible participants must prove they meet federal poverty guidelines and fall beneath a minimum amount of countable assets. Stamps can be used to purchase breads, cereals, produce, meats, dairy products, and seeds or garden plants that produce fruits and vegetables. Stamps may not be used to purchase nonfoods or hot foods.

THE USDA'S MYPLATE

The USDA's Food Pyramid was heavily criticized for being vague and confusing, and in 2011 it was replaced with MyPlate. MyPlate is much easier to understand, as it consists of a picture of a dinner plate divided into four sections, visually illustrating how our daily diet should be distributed among the various food groups. Vegetables and grains each take up 30% of the plate, while fruits and proteins each constitute 20% of the plate. There is also a representation of a cup, marked Dairy, alongside the plate. The idea behind MyPlate is that it's much easier for people to grasp the idea that half of a meal should consist of fruits and vegetables than it is for them to understand serving sizes for all the different kinds of foods they eat on a regular basis.

Most experts consider MyPlate to be a great improvement over the Food Pyramid, but it has still come under criticism from some quarters. Many believe too much emphasis is placed on protein, and some say the dairy recommendation should be eliminated altogether. The Harvard School of Public Health created its own Healthy Eating Plate to address what it sees as shortcomings in MyPlate. Harvard's guide adds healthy plant-based oils to the mix, stresses whole grains instead of merely grains, recommends drinking water or unsweetened coffee or tea instead of milk, and adds a reminder that physical activity is important.

EXPANDED FOOD AND NUTRITION EDUCATION PROGRAM

The EFNEP is federally funded and conducted through the Cooperative Extension Service in every state and US territory. For more than 30 years, EFNEP has been helping families with children learn how to eat healthier meals and snacks, stretch their food dollars, and reduce the risk of foodborne illness. Adults are faced with the challenges of paying rent, utilities, day care, and other daily expenses, and families experience the stress of trying to provide a variety of nutritious foods and maintain healthy diets on limited budgets. EFNEP provides a variety of tools and ideas to help families cut food costs and provide healthy meals and snacks for family members.

Adults enrolled in EFNEP learn how to:

- Plan low-cost nutritious meals.
- Prepare quick and healthy meals and snacks.
- Shop for the best food buys.
- Keep foods safe to eat.
- Eat right and light to control sugar, salt, fat, and calories.

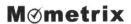

Monitoring and Evaluation

NUTRITION MONITORING

Nutrition monitoring refers to the ongoing process of surveillance of a patient's status by gathering information about the patient's status in relation to their diagnosis, treatment plan, and outcome. Monitoring is important to ascertain whether the patient is improving, or whether corrective action needs to be taken based on lack of progress or failure to meet desired outcomes. Monitoring data should be collected from the initiation of the intervention, and should be reviewed regularly to determine that the activities of the intervention are being transformed into results that meet some specified standard.

MANAGEMENT EVALUATION TOOLS

Nutrition protocols may be developed by a profession or an organization to assist the professionals in making the best decisions for patient care. They may be included in the policy and procedure manual of an organization, so that each clinician follows the same principles of care and service delivery for patients with a particular diagnosis. The protocol reads like a set of instructions, and may include timelines for delivering treatments, monitoring procedures, appropriate lab work, and when consultations should be sought.

Outcome management systems gather data that allow the professional to evaluate the efficacy of an entire process in a timely manner, so that improvements can be made. The data may be compiled in such a way that it is accessible to a number of organizational stakeholders, such as patients, taxpayers, accrediting bodies, or the media. Statistical sampling may be used to evaluate the treatment of large numbers of patients, and results are compared with previous findings or benchmarks of other model organizations.

NUTRITION EVALUATION

Nutrition evaluation is a tool used to measure the efficacy of the nutrition intervention on a patient. The evaluation process measures objective outcomes that show that the patient's behavior or health has improved as a result of the service or intervention. An example would be demonstrating that the diabetic patient can monitor his or her own blood glucose and adjust insulin doses as needed.

INDICATORS

Indicators are used in the quality assurance process as a marker to direct attention to processes or outcomes that need additional investigation. In other words, indicators serve as monitoring tools that allow the professional to monitor the quality of care and make adjustments.

RATE-BASED INDICATORS: Rate-based indicators use data to evaluate what would happen if the best possible care was provided. The indicator is expressed as a rate or proportion. For example, this indicator might ask, "What would happen if 95% of the patients in ABC Nursing Home maintained ideal body weight for a six-month period?" A tolerable threshold would be developed for this nursing home, and any number below the acceptable threshold would be a reason to initiate a plan of action.

SENTINEL EVENT INDICATORS: A sentinel indicator refers to a serious event or incident that would always provide a reason for further action or investigation. The threshold for these incidents is always 0% or 100%. For example, 0% of patients in the nursing home will acquire *Salmonella*.

GUARDING CONSUMERS AGAINST FRAUDULENT CARE

NATIONAL COUNCIL AGAINST HEALTH FRAUD

The National Council Against Health Fraud is a private, voluntary agency that advocates for the consumer by focusing on and identifying the public health problems of quackery and misinformation. They argue that nutrition products and services should be safe and effective, and they believe in the importance of the scientific process for validating claims. They lobby for consumer health laws, investigate claims of dubious health products and services, and educate the public about health fraud through various mechanisms.

FEDERAL TRADE COMMISSION

The Federal Trade Commission (FTC) is the government's agency for protecting consumers. Consumers can file a complaint with the FTC or get free information on issues to help consumers spot and avoid bogus products. They advise that a healthy amount of skepticism be used when evaluating nutritional products such as those that promise easy weight loss.

HIPAA

HIPAA guidelines state the medical documentation entered by a health care provider is considered to be a permanent legal document; as such notes should be typed or written in black ink. Enter notes in the medical chart during or immediately following the visit. All entries should be signed and dated. If an entry has to be made after the interaction with the patient, the time of the interaction and the time the entry was made should be noted.

If diet orders are incorrect in the chart, the dietitian should contact the doctor who wrote the order rather than making the change him or herself. If the dietitian needs to make a correction, the proper procedure is to draw a single line through the text and initial and date the change. If the change is to be made after documentation is complete, an addendum can be added to the chart. Corrections are not to be made by obliterating the original note or by removing pages from the chart.

FEEDBACK SYSTEMS

NEGATIVE FEEDBACK SYSTEM:

"The output reverses the input." The result is to reverse the original change to the controlled condition; if original input was a decrease in activity, then output will be to increase it. Conversely, if original input was an increase in activity, then output will be to decrease it. Another way of stating it is that there is an opposite directional change with negative feedback systems. The result of a negative feedback system should be to maintain the controlled condition within its very narrow, ideal range.

POSITIVE FEEDBACK SYSTEM:

"The output reinforces the input." The result is to strengthen/reinforce the original change to the controlled condition. Since the original input is an increase in activity, then the output will be to increase that activity even further. Another way of stating it is that there is a same directional change with a positive feedback system. The result of a negative feedback system is to make the controlled condition progressively increase.

DOCUMENTATION

HIPAA

HIPAA is the acronym for Health Insurance Portability and Accountability Act. This act became effective in 1996, and it is also known as the Kennedy-Kassebaum Act. The four main objectives of the act are to regulate computer-to-computer sharing of information (the "transaction standard"), provide universal identifiers for healthcare providers and healthcare plans, implement information security regulations, and establish a privacy rule. The privacy rule portion of HIPAA is of particular importance to healthcare providers and, specifically, dietitians as it clearly regulates how medical information is handled, secured, and maintained.

PRIVACY RULE

The privacy rule portion of HIPAA, the Health Insurance Portability and Accountability Act, was instated in 2003, and it specifically deals with a patient's right to privacy in regard to his/her medical care. Upon an initial visit with a medical practitioner, all patients must receive and acknowledge receipt of a privacy notice. The patient's chart must always be handled with the utmost care and confidentiality, such that none other than the patient's care team has access to the information contained within his/her record. All records must be physically secured and/or password protected if electronically documented. Other than the medical team (to include treatment, payment, and healthcare operations personnel), only the patient and his/her designated representative are allowed access to the medical record.

**Note: HIPAA does have additional disclosures that allow access to medical records in the interest of public health, law enforcement, research, government functions, etc.

Principles of Education and Training

Assessment and Planning

MODELS AND THEORIES
CHANGE MODEL

Although individuals may understand the need to adopt healthier lifestyle choices, successful long-term change is difficult to achieve. The stages of the change model argue that behavior change does not happen as a single event; rather, it occurs gradually over time in a recognizable series of steps. In the pre-contemplation stage, the person is not interested in change, and may be in denial regarding serious health issues. When contemplation occurs, the person begins to consider making a change, weighing the pros and cons. During the preparation phase, patients become determined to change, and may try the new behavior in small doses to test the waters. When the action stage is reached, patients adopt the desired behavior. In maintenance, the new behavior becomes ingrained over the long term as a habit. Occasional slip-ups may characterize the maintenance stage. Recognizing which stage an individual is in can help the health professional plan an intervention to help that person move on to the next stage.

HEALTH BELIEF MODEL

The health belief model attempts to explain why individuals choose not to take part in healthy lifestyle changes or programs designed to improve their health, even when the person knows he or she is at risk for illness or disability due to health status. The model presents several belief and value continuums that predict whether change will occur. Perceived susceptibility describes how likely a person feels he or she is to experience disease or adverse effects. Perceived seriousness refers to the extent the person believes the disease or problem would affect his or her life. A perceived benefit of action implies that the person recognizes the disease possibility as serious, and is weighing the benefits of change. Barriers to taking action may include negative beliefs about change or physical or social impediments to change. Cues to action may be external, from a family member or health professional, or internal messages prompting change.

DIFFUSION OF INNOVATION THEORY

Diffusion of innovation is a theory that attempts to explain how new behaviors or innovations spread through a population. Innovators are the first to adopt the new idea or behavior, and they are characterized as risk-taking and open to change. Early adopters are people who are respected by members of their group, and can be influential in speeding up the diffusion process. The early majority follows, and adopts the new idea or behavior just before the rest of the group. The late majority is more skeptical to the newness of the idea, and may not adopt the new behavior until peer pressure causes them to relent. The laggards care little about the opinions and behaviors of others, preferring to remain in their comfort zone. In some populations, targeting the opinion leaders can provide a shortcut to gaining compliance in the rest of the population.

BLOOM'S TAXONOMY

Bloom's taxonomy argues that there are multiple learning styles, and this can be helpful to recognize before preparing educational nutritional programs. The cognitive domain can be understood in terms of the acquisition of knowledge. This type of learning would include recalling facts, such as being able to explain the different levels in the food pyramid. Comprehension is also a part of cognitive learning, and getting someone to describe the healthy fats in his or her own words can show comprehension. The affective domain encompasses one's attitudes and emotions about

59

the subject material. The willingness to listen respectfully and respond to questions asked by the discussion leader is an example of affective learning. The formation of values regarding the learning material also falls in the affective realm, such as when the individual changes his or her schedule to make time to prepare healthy meals. Psychomotor learning can be thought of in terms of skills gained. The ability to check one's blood glucose is an accomplishment of psychomotor learning.

BEHAVIOR MODIFICATION

The psychologist B.F. Skinner argued that the environment was more important in shaping behavior than one's thought processes. He said that people's behavior can be predicted through the observation of stimuli and responses. Skinner said that because the stimulus is not always present to cause a behavior, the result of the behavior is more important than the presence of the stimulus. If an individual expects a positive result, he or she will engage in the behavior. If a negative result is expected, the behavior will be avoided. When the positive result is achieved repeatedly, this provides positive reinforcement.

Modeling refers to the behavior change that occurs when an individual copies the behavior displayed by another person, the model. If the model possesses characteristics the observer values, such as power or intelligence, the observer will be more likely to imitate the behavior. Targeting highly respected members of a population can prepare them to serve as models for the rest of the population.

Avoidance learning occurs when an individual learns to behave in a certain way in order to avoid unpleasant consequences. The behavior is reinforced by the individual's desire to avoid the punishment. An example of this is in a case of nutritional counseling, where an individual is chastised by a health professional because he or she is not following his or her prescribed renal diet, resulting in further kidney problems. The individual follows the diet, not because of the kidney problems, but because he or she wants to avoid further criticism.

Extinction learning is often discussed in the context of fear conditioning. If an unpleasant stimulus is paired with a neutral stimulus, eventually the neutral stimulus will elicit a response. Then, when the neutral stimulus is presented alone, eventually the fear response will be eliminated.

Punishment involves trying to change behavior by providing an unpleasant consequence as a result of the behavior. If the punishment occurs repeatedly, learned helplessness occurs, where the individual feels the problem has no solution.

EDUCATIONAL NEEDS ASSESSMENT

In order to develop appropriate educational interventions, it is necessary to assess the needs and readiness to learn of the intended audience or population. One should assess how motivated the target audience is to learn. Highly motivated individuals may be very interested in the topic and will attend counseling sessions whether they are mandatory or not, while those with low motivation will feel the education is not useful to him or her. Educational level should be assessed to plan the most effective teaching style. An audience with a high level of education can understand complex messages, while those with a low level of education need simple messages and benefit from repetition. Level of sophistication may tie in with education. Highly sophisticated people may already consider themselves self-styled experts in the field; those with little sophistication include children or those never exposed to nutrition messages before. Socioeconomic status should also be considered. Upper income adults tend to be more interested in health foods. Poor individuals are focused on coping with immediate problems.

60

COMMUNITY NUTRITION PROGRAMS

When developing a nutrition program geared toward a specific population, the first step is to develop a mission statement, or the guiding philosophy of the program. Defining the needs of the population is central in forming this philosophy. Next, one should define some broad goals that the program is meant to achieve. The next step is to hone in on the goals to formulate some measurable objectives that give meaning and purpose to the program; these should be written as concrete action statements. Then one should define the focus of the program by setting priorities; this may mean that some goals will need to be set aside. With prioritized goals in place one can develop a plan of action, which should include all of the alternative ways of achieving the goals. A budget can then be developed, and implementation of the plan follows. Depending on the scope of the program, implementation may include small-scale outreach efforts like health fairs or may involve lobbying to pass new legislation.

EDUCATIONAL PROGRAMS

DESIGN AND DEVELOPMENT

The development of a solid educational plan begins with an analysis of the existing information. The material should be matched to the objectives the instructor wants to achieve, and the information should be organized in a logical fashion that complements the retention of the material. A detailed lesson plan should include a summary of each section, the time set aside for each lesson, and the formative and summative assessment tools that will be used. Learning should have everyday applications in order to bring the subject matter to life. Quality visual aids such as posters or power point presentations make the presentation more engaging. In some cases, short video presentations may be appropriate to supplement the instructor's lessons.

COMMUNICATION PRINCIPLES

Good nutritional instruction requires excellent communication and critical thinking skills. Establishing rapport with the client allows him or her to share anxieties about lifestyle changes, and lets the instructor know where to focus his or her support. Even small changes in lifestyle can seem overwhelming to the client, so offering as many alternatives as possible to give control back to the client can help to reduce fears. Empathizing with the client can help build rapport by allowing the client to feel understood. The educational message should be clear but not rigid. Including the client in the learning process also empowers the client and can enhance retention of knowledge. Good listening skills include paraphrasing the client's message or asking for clarification to reduce ambiguity. Soliciting feedback from the client can help the instructor tailor the message and teaching method as the learning continues.

GROUP DYNAMICS PRINCIPLES

Providing good leadership when conducting a group counseling session can help propel the group towards its goals smoothly. Groups are by nature inclusive, so the leader should promote group harmony and make everyone feel accepted. Skillful leaders do not monopolize the interactions; rather, they make suggestions or offer ideas to facilitate discussion, and then wait patiently for the group to converse. However, if the conversation wanders off topic or exchanges become heated, the leader should step in to resume control. The leader may involve non-participants in a tactful way, without putting them on the spot. Sometimes it may be necessary to wrest control away from an overly dominating member. Praise should be offered equally, so that no one feels silenced because one member is favored over another. It is helpful to have an agenda planned in advance; organization keeps the control with the leader and thus reduces the opportunity for conflict.

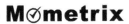

TEACHING METHODS

Large group instruction is appropriate when a clear, unambiguous message needs to be relayed to a large group of people without the need for much discussion. Examples include conferences, where professionals are usually speaking to their peers, and lectures, where groups of students are taking in a great deal of subject matter in an abbreviated period. Small group discussion is beneficial when a group of several people have similar backgrounds. In this setting the lecture is interspersed with frequent discussion, which allows the participants to learn from and support one another. Self-paced instruction is usually computer-based, such as a web-based module that a health professional completes for continuing education credits. This form of learning is better for the highly motivated and educated learner. Question-answer techniques place a high value on student participation. Examples include role-play, which stimulates thought about real life implications of the materials. Focused recitation uses class discussion to arrive at a solution or answer to a problem under the guidance of the instructor. The solution has been preordained, but the creative process of brainstorming and working together gives the students ownership of the problem and improves the retention of knowledge. Guided practice involves allowing the students to try a new skill under the tutelage of the instructor before returning home to try the skill alone. An example is a healthy cooking class where the dietitian guides the students as they prepare low fat, high flavor dishes. Role-playing helps the student become more comfortable with an upcoming lifestyle change by pretending to adopt the behavior with a classmate acting in a supporting role. For example, a child preparing to go on dialysis may act out the process with a peer, which can reduce anxiety about the procedure. The teacher provides feedback and uses the dialogue to further the discussion.

ASSESSMENTS

Formative assessment is conducted throughout the educational process. The goal of formative assessment is to discover what the target group knows and what they do not understand, so that teaching methods can be tailored throughout the duration of teaching. Encouraging frequent discussion among participants can give the instructor cues that reveal what topics are still unclear to the individual. Breaking into small groups for discussion, and then sharing those thoughts with the larger group can also provide insight to the instructor. Frequent, brief quizzes may also communicate where learning gaps lie.

Summative assessments include the typical final exams or tests that evaluate how well one has learned the material as a whole. This kind of assessment is more formalized, as opposed to the informal discussions that can characterize formative assessments. Although summative assessments cannot help the instructor change the learning that has already taken place, they may help identify areas for improvement in future educational endeavors.

SUCCESSFUL INTERVIEWS

In the context of patient counseling, the interview is a chance to obtain complete information from the patient about his or her eating habits, and it can reveal other social, cultural, environmental, or socio-economic issues that will affect the patient's willingness or ability to take part in the counseling. The first step is to collect factual data, such as age, weight, and height, giving the client time to become comfortable with the interview process. Open-ended questions are important, as this gives the patient opportunity to expand upon their answer and provide information the interviewer might not otherwise have received. Instead of, "Are you watching your fat grams?" say, "Describe your typical breakfast/lunch/dinner." If the client pauses frequently, avoid leading them to an answer in order to move the interview along. Summarize what you heard and noted at the end of the interview to give the client a chance to correct any errors, and tell him or her how you will use the information that was gathered.

LEARN

The LEARN framework is a five-step plan that can improve the communication between a clinician and a patient so that the implementation of the treatment plan will go smoothly. The first step is to use active listening skills and attend to the patient's concerns with empathy. Putting oneself in the shoes of the patient can facilitate understanding. The second step is to explain one's perception of the problem, or to justify one's opinions about the situation to the patient. Using "I" statements instead of "you" statements will avoid putting the patient on the defense. The third step is to acknowledge and discuss differences. This should be done with empathy, for example, "I can understand why you are anxious about this change, but this is why it is so important to your health." The fourth step is to recommend the appropriate treatment. The last step is to negotiate treatment, or reach a middle ground where the patient agrees to participate at a level satisfactory to both patient and clinician.

Implementation and Evaluation

PATIENT EDUCATION

The effectiveness of nutritional education is largely dependent upon the delivery of that information. First, consider the audience—will information be delivered to children, adults, or the elderly? Does the individual have the cognitive ability to digest the information? Consider the attention span and energy level of the individual and attempt to counsel him/her during his/her most alert part of the day. Next, prepare the information in a manner suitable to the individual's learning style. Always leave notes and/or a pamphlet of information behind. Counsel the individual in regards to his/her dietary limitations, necessary changes, deficiencies, etc. Provide tools and motivation for the individual to make the necessary changes. Make suggestions to enhance long-term outcomes. It is important that emphasis be placed on the need for change. If the client does not understand the need for dietary change, the nutritional education will be for naught.

NUTRITIONAL EDUCATION RESOURCES

There are many resources available to individuals wishing to change their eating habits. Resources are available in the community and virtually. Some of those resources include:

Virtual Resources	Community Resources
Mypyramid.gov	Home healthcare agencies
American Heart Association website	Local nursing associations
American Cancer Society website	Local dietary associations
American Diabetes Association website	Meals on Wheels
American Dietetics Association website	Senior Services/Centers
USDA website	

TEACHING PORTION SIZE

When educating a client in regards to portion size, it is helpful to provide everyday comparisons, or models, for portion size. This allows a client to more adequately "eyeball" the correct portion size. Some common comparison models are as follows:

- Meat, 1 oz. = Matchbox
- Meat, poultry, 3 oz. (typical serving size) = Deck of cards or palm of hand
- Cheese, 1 oz = 4 dice
- Potato, medium = Computer mouse
- Peanut butter, 2 Tbsp = Ping pong or golf ball

63

- Pasta, ice cream, ½ cup = Tennis ball or a cupped hand
- Bagel = Hockey puck
- Fruits/Vegetables = Baseball
- Pancake/Waffle = CD
- Fish, 3 oz. = Checkbook

DETERMINING PATIENT INTEREST

There are many cues that may indicate an individual's interest to learn new material. Some of those are evident by body language. An individual who looks eager often is. Eagerness may be indicated by attention to the speaker/counselor, interest in taking notes, making eye contact, asking questions, welcoming the individual, and other similar cues. On the other hand, someone with crossed arms, avoiding eye contact, appearing tired or uninterested, and/or changing the subject may not be ready to discuss any topic, let alone a topic regarding nutritional education. Additionally, ask the individual if s/he is motivated to make dietary changes. If the client responds positively, then begin the conversation. Finally, note whether the client is inquisitive either verbally or non-verbally.

DISCERNING PATIENT UNDERSTANDING

Patient understanding is paramount to proper treatment and therapy. It is important, therefore, to determine whether an individual understands received counseling and nutritional education. Evaluate the level of a patient's understanding by asking the patient questions about topics discussed. Additionally, ask the patient if s/he can and will recap the discussion and/or action plan set forth. Moreover, the educator may also ask if the patient has any questions and what those questions are. It is appropriate to lead the patient to ask specific questions that will direct the discussion to key points of the educational session.

**Note: It is always appropriate and prudent to leave printed educational materials for further review and for patient reference.

INCORPORATING SELECTIVE MENUS

Selective menus are designed to aid patients in healthy food choices. These particular menus allow patients a choice of menu items that when combined provide a well-balanced meal. By allowing patients to choose menu items, the facility is essentially granting greater patient autonomy. Additionally, patients consistently see healthy menus, comprised of items that, taken in whole, make a well-balanced meal. Therefore, patients learn through the use of a directed example how to pair menu items to create healthy meals. Not only are the patients learning how to create a well-balanced meal, but they are also being directed towards healthy foods and away from high-fat, high-sugar sources. Additionally, proper portion sizes of the menu items will further enforce healthy eating habits.

HELPFUL LEARNING TOOLS

Various materials may be helpful in imparting nutritional education to clients. The type of materials may be determined by age, ailment afflicting patients, and type of information to be conveyed to the patients. Some helpful materials are listed below.

- Pamphlets and brochures recapping information. Be sure to have large-print, Braille, and picture pamphlets handy.
- Food models and portion size comparison models, including a deck of cards, balls of various sizes (tennis, ping pong, golf ball, etc.), dice, matchbooks, and modeling with client's hand.
- Pictures and graphics of plates representing well-balanced meals, personalized food plan.

- Exchange diet equivalents.
- Diagram explaining how to read/dissect nutritional facts labeling information.
- Computer-generated aging programs, if available.

MAXIMIZING THE EFFECTIVENESS OF WRITTEN MATERIALS

Written materials are essential elements of patient education as they serve as a source of reference outside of dietary counseling sessions. Patients with impaired memory, who experience difficulty concentrating, and/or are suffering from fatigue may rely on written materials to guide their nutritional choices. The most effective written materials are printed in an easy to read font, that is both stylistically simplistic and of adequate size. Capitalization and punctuation should be properly utilized. Additionally, the materials should be kept as simple as possible, minimizing the use of complex sentences, large words, vocabulary consisting of medical and/or scientific jargon, and inclusion of excessive information. Spacing between lines and paragraphs should be such that the information may be easily read. Graphics and/or diagrams may be used to help explain topics, though excessive use of pictures may detract from the message being conveyed.

DIETARY COUNSELING
STRUCTURING DIETARY COUNSELING

It is important that dietary counseling/education be methodically prepared and presented. In order to do so, the client's health and dietary needs are first *assessed* by the dietary manager and the patient's care team. After the assessment, a plan with future dietary changes and goals must be *developed* and followed. In order for the plan to be *implemented,* the developed plan must be realistic in its expectations. Finally, ongoing evaluations must be performed in order to ensure that the needs found by the assessment are, in fact, being addressed by the developed plan and implemented by the patient and care team. An evaluation of the plan may be used to revise dietary goals and plan expectations.

CUSTOMIZING A NUTRITIONAL COUNSELING SESSION

It is crucial that nutritional counseling be tailored to the individual, as each person has specific and unique needs. Even among individuals prescribed the same diets, it is imperative that each person receives specialized and individual counseling. Elements of counseling should include information about the patient's nutritional needs and restrictions, which should be personalized based upon the individual's taste preferences, regional recipes, and religious and/or cultural observances. Additionally, learning materials, including visual aids, videos, food portion models, and other similar tools should also be tailored to the individual being counseled. An individual with impaired vision, for example, should be provided large print reading materials and/or audio notes. Finally, take into account any adaptive equipment that an individual may use during mealtime. The adaptive equipment may influence the individual's willingness and ability to eat certain items. Patients may also need to be taught how to effectively utilize adaptive equipment.

PROVEN COUNSELING TECHNIQUES

Various counseling techniques may be used to convey nutritional information, implement a healthy program, and set goals for future progress. Some of the following techniques may be helpful:

- Assess whether the patient is ready and motivated to make behavior changes and modification. If so, proceed with nutritional counseling. If not, it is imperative that the counselor impresses upon the client the need for change. If the individual is not willing to make changes, further counseling will be for naught.

- Help the client set realistic goals. If the client feels empowered, s/he is more apt to reach his/her goals. Setting goals for the client may undermine the counseling and his/her motivation to change.
- Ask the patient if s/he feels comfortable involving a support system. If so, bring these individuals into counseling to help "check" and motivate the patient when s/he needs it.
- Stress the importance of keeping an accurate journal, to include information about food, biological markers (including blood glucose measurements, if necessary), and emotions about food and/or goals.

CHARACTERISTICS OF EFFECTIVE COMMUNICATION

Effective communication is evidenced by mutual understanding, body language, and follow-through on information discussed. Some characteristics of effective communication include the following:

- *Good eye contact.* Eye contact shared by both parties conveys interest and understanding between the individuals. Looking down or away from the presenter may indicate that a topic is not well understood, is an uncomfortable subject, or needs further discussion.
- *Effective oral communication.* When communicating orally, it is imperative that all parties understand one another. Slow, clear speech greatly improves understanding and comprehension of material discussed. Additionally, hearing devices and/or translators should be used when necessary.
- *Open dialogue.* Even when presenting nutritional information to another, an open dialogue is important. Questions asked to and from both individuals helps drive critical points and clarify weakly communicated topics.
- *Quiet, undisturbed environment.* Communication in any counseling setting is most effective in a quiet environment with little distraction.

FRIENDS AND FAMILY

Friends and family are an integral part of counseling as they are often the most influential forces in a patient's life. Family may be able to encourage and motivate a client to make changes to his/her diet, and in effect, improve the health of the patient. Additionally, family members and friends may be willing to modify their diet in order to follow the nutritional guidelines set forth for the patient. Friends and family are also a great source of accountability for patients. Not only can these individuals help the patient stay on his/her nutritional plan, but these individuals may also assist in dietary journaling/documentation. This is especially important when the patient has dementia or impaired memory.

Foodservice Systems

Menu Planning

FEDERAL REGULATIONS

Federal regulations mandate that all facilities provide their clients with nourishing, palatable food that is presented as part of a well-balanced diet. Menus must satisfy total nutritional needs, be palatable and attractively presented. Additionally, a menu plan must be prepared in advance and followed. The food on the plan must be properly prepared and served at a healthy temperature. Moreover, the food and/or menu must be adapted for patients' individual needs. Patients who refuse food must be offered a substitute that has an equivalent nutritive value. Physician prescribed therapeutic diets must be followed. Finally, facilities must have at least three scheduled mealtimes, at regular intervals throughout the day. There may be no more than fourteen hours between a dinner meal and breakfast meal, except in the case where a nutritive snack is offered, in which the interval between those meals may be stretched to sixteen hours.

Federal regulations mandate that care facilities provide appropriate feeding assistive devices (lip plate, weighted utensils, cups, feeding devices, and others) and feeding staff where necessary. Paid staff that assists with feedings must work under the supervision of a licensed or registered nurse and must be trained. Training should be comprised of a minimum of eight hours of education on the following topics: feeding and hydration techniques and assistance, communication and behavioral response, safety procedures (to include the Heimlich maneuver), infection control, resident rights, and patient monitoring (so that an assistant may properly note and report any behavioral changes displayed by the client). These assistants are not allowed to feed patients with complicated feeding problems, to include those who have difficulty swallowing, have persistent/reoccurring aspiration of the lungs, and/or must be fed intravenously or through the use of a tube.

POSTED MENU REGULATIONS

Federal regulations mandate that menus not only be followed, but that they are prepared in advance and in accordance to the recommendations of the Food and Nutrition Board of the National Research Council, National Academy of Sciences. Deviation from the posted menu is only allowed in the cases where a client refuses food. In such cases, a menu substitute may be offered as long as it has similar nutritional value to the posted menu item. In addition to federal regulations regarding posted menus, facilities must also follow any regulations mandated by the state in which the facility operates. As law is continuously evolving, it is important to review state and federal law regularly to ensure compliance.

SERVING SIZES

Though often used interchangeably, portion size and serving size are not necessarily equivalent amounts of food. Portion size is the amount of food that one serves and consumes. Thus, portion size may vary from person to person. On the contrary, serving size refers to the amount of food to which the nutritional values refer. A serving size may or may not match the recommended portion size of a food. For example, if one were to compare the serving size of various cereals, he might find that one brand recommends a serving size of three-quarters of a cup whereas another brand may recommend a serving size of one cup. The nutritional values reflect the fat, calorie, and vitamin content of one serving.

ADA SERVING SIZES

The American Dietetic Association (ADA) recommends modest portion sizes, equivalent to the below serving sizes.

- Meat, 3 ounces
- Margarine, 1 teaspoon
- Pasta, 1 cup
- Cheese, 1 ½ ounces
- Bread, 1 slice or 1 ounce
- Bagel, ½ medium
- Peanut butter, 2 tablespoons
- Milk, 1 cup
- Vegetables, ½ cup

PORTIONING

Proper portioning of food results in less waste and helps to control costs. Therefore, it is important that the proper portions of food are served. Proper portioning must also be done quickly to ensure temperature and taste quality of food as well as cost-effectiveness. It is advisable to use standardized food service tools such as scoops, ladles, and dishers to ensure correct portioning. Additionally, servers should cut batches into the number of servings indicated by yield, such that a pie meant to serve six is, in fact, cut into six equal pieces or a loaf of bread designed to provide 20 slices is sliced in that manner. Using correct pan sizes also ensures proper portioning.

Listed below are the size numbers and equivalent measures of standardized scoops.

#6 = 2/3 cup
#8 = ½ cup
#10 = 3/8 cup
#12 = 1/3 cup
#16 = ¼ cup
#20 = 3 1/3 tablespoon
#24 = 2 2/3 tablespoon
#30 = 2 tablespoon
#40 = 1 2/3 tablespoon
#50 = 3 ¾ teaspoon
#60 = 3 ¼ teaspoon
#70 = 2 ¾ teaspoon
#100 = 2 teaspoon

RECIPES

A standardized recipe is a recipe that has been tried and modified multiple times. Once the recipe meets taste and quality standards, the process is written out such that any food service employee should be able to make the recipe and produce the same results as any other food service employee. Additionally, the yield of the recipe should be equal regardless of who prepares the recipe, provided that they directly follow the written process. A standardized recipe's process should include information regarding the exact measurements of ingredients, the order that the ingredients are added to one another, and information on how to properly mix those ingredients. Additionally, a standardized recipe will include information about how to properly cook the item being served.

A standardized recipe is essential to menu planning for a variety of reasons. Some of those reasons include:

- The recipe produces a consistent yield, which ensures enough food will be made.
- Every serving of the recipe will have an equal nutritional composition—regardless of when it is prepared or who it is prepared by.
- Standardized recipes allow for more effective menu planning and food purchasing.
- Food preparation time can be accurately gauged when using a standardized recipe.
- A standardized recipe will result in the same product, each time it is made. Therefore, tastes, texture, and color can all be anticipated.

ELEMENTS

As a standardized recipe is used to promote consistency, it is not surprising then that every standardized recipe should contain some key elements. Those elements include:

- Name of recipe; name should be unique and descriptive.
- Recipe category and number (if the organization uses a number system).
- Recipe yield.
- Serving size (this is what will make the yield consistent).
- Food ingredients.
- Food safety information.
- Directions for mixing.
- Pan size, shape, and material.
- Bake time and temperature.
- Serving utensils.

SAMPLE CATEGORIES FOR RECIPES

It is important that recipes be organized in a manner that is convenient and easily understood. Recipes may be organized into categories based upon the primary ingredient, so that categories may include: meats, seafood, poultry, vegetables, fruits, and others. Recipes may also be organized by the type of dish, such that categories may include: entrees, appetizers, vegetables, fruits, beverages, desserts, breads, and other categories. Or, recipes may be organized in a manner that combines the main ingredient with the type of dish, such that category offerings may include: beef entrees, poultry entrees, seafood entrees, vegetarian entrees, cake desserts, pie and pastry desserts, etc. Regardless of the method adopted by a specific organization, recipe categorization should be consistent and according to the organization's adopted policy.

HOW TO SCALE A RECIPE

Recipe scaling is integral to cooking enough food but minimizing waste. Scaling is the act of adjusting a recipe to meet the organization's needs. In some cases, scaling means cutting a recipe down and in others, it means increasing the recipe's unit of production. The following example shows how to scale a recipe (that typically yields 8 portions) to feed 214 people. Divide the number of servings needed by the number of servings yielded in each batch. So, $(214)/(8) = 26.75$

Depending upon the type of recipe, you may choose to round up to the nearest whole number. For example, one cannot easily make ¾ of a cake, so the recipe would be rounded up such that 27 batch units would be made. All ingredient amounts in the recipe would need to be multiplied by 27. Cooking/baking times might also need adjustment.

Generally speaking, it is advisable to convert measurements of ingredients from volume measurements to weight prior to scaling. This is done for multiple reasons, primary of which is ease of use. When using volume measurements, one may be dealing with multiple fractions, which makes math more difficult. Moreover, measuring by weight is often quicker when making a large recipe than measuring by volume. Keep in mind that when scaling recipes, it may not be necessary to precisely scale all ingredients. Some ingredients such as butter and oil used for sautéing, spices, frostings, and others may be needed in smaller quantities than scaling might indicate.

CONTROLLING COSTS

The most effective way to control costs when using a standardized recipe is to follow the recipe exactly as it is written and to scale the recipe ONLY to the number of servings needed. If, for example, a cook added more meat than what was required by a recipe to avoid measuring out pre-packaged meat, the cost per serving of the meal just increased. Moreover, if an item is not properly cut into portions equaling the specified serving size, the recipe may become more costly. Larger portions result in fewer servings, which increase the cost per serving. If extra-large portions are consistently served, a large portion of the kitchen budget may quickly disappear.

FORECASTING

Forecasting in food services is just like weather forecasting; it is the process of predicting future needs, to include future inventory needs (and thus, purchasing needs) as well as service needs (number of portions, types of items). When forecasting, it is important to have the following types of records on-hand: previous census records, tallies, points-of-sale, and special orders/special diets. Forecasting requires knowledge of previous menus, inventories and purchases to help shape future food service needs. For example, if, in the past, portion sizes were made smaller than the suggested serving size to feed the number of people needing meals, it is helpful to have that information as direction to order additional food ingredients. Additionally, if there was excess waste in the past, it may be advisable to decrease the purchase order and/or to serve a different item.

SEQUENCING

The sequence in which food is prepared, from ordering to thawing, preparing, cooking, and serving is very important for a variety of reasons. First, one must ensure that all items are on-hand and available for a planned menu. The food items must then be thawed (if necessary) such that the items are ready to be cooked but not so far in advance that the item spoils. In addition to individual food item preparatory sequencing, it is also important that a meal, as a whole follows proper sequencing, such that food items are cooked and ready for service at approximately the same time. If for example, roast beef, mashed potatoes, and salad were on a dinner menu, and all were to be served at the same time, but the roast beef was finished before the salads were prepared, the meat would cool prior to service. If, instead, the meat was prepared and left to slow cook while the salad was being prepared, the items would be finished at similar times and both would be presented at an acceptable temperature, without wilting.

CYCLE MENUS

A cycle menu is one where different menus are planned for each day over a specified period of time. At the end of that period, the entire cycle menu is repeated. A cycle may take as few as three to four days or may be as long as a couple of months. When used correctly, a cycle menu allows food service personnel to more effectively order food and prepare meals. Because the overall menu is repeated, the kitchen staff may more easily anticipate food, time, and labor needs. Additionally, clients know what to expect of the menu and may look forward to certain meals.

A cycle menu runs the risk of becoming too repetitive, which may result in clients becoming bored with the menu. For this reason, longer cycles are preferable to shorter ones. Additionally, when utilizing a cycle menu, it is advisable to avoid matching menu items to certain days of the week. For example, offering pasta on Monday, chicken on Tuesday, and so on, every week, only emphasizes the repetitive nature of the menu. If, instead, one matches menu items to Day 1, Day 2, and so on, and if the cycle is not repeated every seven days, the menu will appear to be much less repetitive to many clients.

CLIENT ACCEPTANCE

PRESENTATION

Simple touches can make dining much more attractive to clients. Some of those touches include:

- Fill the plate with a variety of color. Pair brightly colored fruits and vegetables with meats, poultry, and fish.
- Use fresh herbs as garnish. Drizzle or pipe sauces on foods rather than pouring or ladling sauces.
- Consider purchasing two coordinating sets of tableware. A change in plate color may make food pop. Additionally, tables may be set with a combination of the sets.
- Add flowers to the table. Use a variety of colored table linens. Ensure linens are clean and without stains.
- Serve food quickly to prevent "wilting" of meats, fruits, and vegetables or "cooking" of items left on heat plates.
- Do not overcook food. Again, the appearance of dried or "wilted" food is unappetizing.
- Make the tables and menu items easily available to everyone. Have adequate space for wheelchairs and adaptive equipment.

Individuals will naturally be more excited to eat when the dining facility and food presented look appealing. Appetizing presentation is particularly important in long-term care facilities where many patients are often suffering from some type of vitamin/mineral deficiency, malnourishment, and depression. Careful and colorful arrangement of food on a plate may entice customers to not only eat but also to try all of the menu items. Thus, if menus are planned correctly, clients have a greater chance of consuming a well-balanced meal. Mealtime is also the perfect time to meet others and pry patients away from the isolation of their rooms. Thus, a pleasurable dining experience will serve patients on a physical, emotional, and social level.

PLATE WASTE

Plate waste is the amount of food left uneaten on a plate by a client. Waste is estimated by comparing the portion size to the amount of food remaining on the plate. It is important to note plate waste, as it is a good indicator of client preferences. If a served menu item consistently results in a large amount of plate waste, it is likely that the clients do not prefer that item. Additionally, if a menu item is often well received but on one occasion results in an abnormally large plate waste, the food may not have been properly prepared, served, and/or was not the correct temperature. On the other hand, if a menu item does not consistently result in plate waste that is a good indicator that the menu item is well received by the institution's clients.

FOOD ACCEPTANCE SURVEYS

A food acceptance survey assists a dietary manager in soliciting the opinions of his/her customer. This survey should include questions regarding food temperature, tastes, attractiveness, portion size, and other factors. Feedback from the survey should be addressed by the dietary staff, and it is advisable to form an advisory panel of staff, customers, and, in the case of a long-term care facility, patient families, that follows up the survey with discussion of the results as well as problem-solving brainstorms. When designing a food acceptance survey, it is important to be as specific as possible without leading clients. Vague questions will solicit vague answers, which may cause frustration when attempting to improve/revise current service. Dissatisfaction expressed via the survey should be directly addressed by investigating alternative cooking and serving methods, changing menu items, utilizing different ingredients, performing tray-line efficiency studies, etc.

SPECIAL NOURISHMENTS

Special nourishments are commonly called:

- Nutritional supplements
- Medical food
- Food for special diets
- Oral supplements
- Liquid meals
- Medical supplements

Special nourishments may be orally, enterally or parenterally consumed. The name of the nourishment may or may not reflect the manner in which it is administered to the patient.

IDENTIFYING PATIENT NEEDS

Special nourishments are most often administered to patients who are malnourished, lose at least five percent of body weight in a month's time, are unable to consume solid or pureed diets, have a specific medical condition that makes it difficult for the individual to swallow, digest, or process food, or those with severely progressed dementia. The decision to prescribe special nourishments should be made by an interdisciplinary team that takes into account a patient's total wellness—physical, emotional, and psychological-- as well as all of the patient's limitations. Patient conditions may digress such that s/he moves from a regular, balanced diet, to a pureed diet, to enteral feedings, and then, parenteral feedings. Additionally, a patient may receive supplemental nourishment even when able to consume food orally.

SUPPLEMENTS

The appropriateness of a supplemental product relies on several factors. Those factors include:

- Ability of the supplement to meet all of the nutritional needs. Supplemental nourishment may need to provide a boost of certain nutrients, minerals, or elements of food. Alternatively, special nourishment may need to provide total nourishment for a client.
- Compatibility with any dietary restrictions brought about by allergy or disease.
- Cost and availability of product.
- Safety of product from production to intake.
- Life of product and suspected length of time nourishment will be needed.

When preparing supplements, great care must be taken to ensure patient health. Proper sanitation (to include hand washing, utilizing sanitized cooking/preparation equipment, and properly cleansing feeding devices) is paramount. Because many patients receiving supplemental nourishment are receiving the food via a tube or IV and because those patients are often already weak, they are at greater risk of infection. Additionally, care should be taken to ensure that the nourishment conforms to the prescribed diet. Because each client's supplement should be prepared specifically for him/her, it is essential to check the supplement against the individual's therapeutic diet.

MENU MODIFICATION

There are many available resources to aid in menu modification. Those resources include:

Facility Dietary Manual. This should be the primary resource when modifying a diet, as it will list commonly used substitutions, facility standards and limitations.

- American Dietetic Association
- American Heart Association
- American Diabetes Association
- American Cancer Society
- National Institutes of Health
- Advocate organizations for specific diseases
- Books addressing specific aging, disease, etc.

Menu modifications may be necessary for a variety of reasons. Some of those reasons may include:

- Physical limitations of the client, for example, an inability to properly chew and swallow food.
- Limitations imposed by a disease and/or gastrointestinal intolerance for or allergy to specific foods.
- Change in health status, to include weight gain or loss or nutrient deficiency.
- Preparation or recovery from a surgery, illness, or gastrointestinal irritation.
- Dementia, which impairs ability to feed oneself or memory to do so.
- Taste aversions and refusal to eat certain foods.
- Religious or ethnic restrictions.

FINGER-FOODS

As a patient's age and/or health declines, they may adapt to preserve their quality of life. One such adaptation is to eat using one's fingers. A patient may do this because of the lack of strength in the upper extremities or because coordination has deteriorated. In such cases, menu modification may be necessary. Small dietary modifications, such as serving chicken strips instead of whole chicken breasts, crudités in place of salad, and cookies or cupcakes in lieu of cakes may be helpful. Additionally, liquid items, such as soups and ice cream, may be served in an easily held cup. Slight menu modifications allow the patient to maintain quality of life and dignity. However, it is important that the patient be frequently monitored for additional changes to ensure adequate nourishment.

MAKING FOOD SUBSTITUTIONS

Patient preference is important to ensuring consumption of a well-balanced meal. Selective menus are helpful in melding both patient preference and providing an equal distribution of vitamins and minerals. When substituting menu items, it is important that menu items of similar or equal nutritional value are substituted. Typically, fruits and vegetables of similar color or structure may be substituted for each other. Often times, poultry may be substituted for other meats. In some cases, nutritional supplements may need to be administered to patients who consistently refuse to eat certain types of food groups. The primary objective, in all cases, is to provide the patient with a well-balanced diet.

COMMON EXCHANGE DIET PORTIONS

Exchange diets are specifically formulated to direct patients with diabetes to eat a healthy diet that regulates carbohydrate intake. Below are the portion equivalents to one exchange:

- Bread, 1 ounce
- Cooked pastas, cereals, grains, ½ cup
- Meat (cooked), 1 ounce
- Vegetables (raw), 1 cup
- Vegetables (cooked), ½ cup
- Vegetables (juiced), ½ cup
- Milk, 1 cup
- Fats, 1 teaspoon

SPEECH THERAPIST ASSISTANCE

Speech therapists are trained to evaluate swallowing and feeding disorders as well as speech disorders. Because feeding and swallowing involve the tongue, mouth, pharynx, larynx, and esophagus (all of which influence one's ability to speak), speech therapists are proficient at working with clients to improve swallowing ability. Therapy is meant to improve dysphagia (difficulty swallowing) by determining the precise mechanism that is hindered or failing. Speech therapists may recommend the use of enteral feeding products either as a means of nourishing a client during therapy, with a goal of tube removal or may recommend enteral feedings when therapy does not remedy the dysphagia.

Procurement and Supply Management

FOOD COST AND QUALITY

While cost often reflects food quality, cost and quality are not always synonymous. Food producers and manufacturers employ a variety of methods for determining cost. It may be dependent upon the quality of food, extent of packaging, expense of transportation, or amount of food purchased at once. It is always important to evaluate the quality of food prior to purchasing. Additionally, a food acceptance survey may be used as a tool for selecting brands based upon client desires. However, be careful to include only affordable brands on the food acceptance survey.

EQUIPMENT
CAPITAL EQUIPMENT

Capital equipment is defined as equipment essential to the function of a job that is usually characterized by an expensive price tag and a long life. So, for example, an appliance such as a meat slicer, refrigerator, or microwave may be classified as capital equipment. Each facility should define "expensive;" some organizations define items priced at $500 or more capital equipment, while others put a higher or lower price on capital equipment. Regardless of the organization's price definition, capital equipment typically needs to be approved before purchase. The process of purchasing such equipment should include: establishing a need, determining whether money is available in the budget, shopping for vendors, models, and prices, asking for the opinions of others within the organization, and preparing a document justifying the purchase. Then, the financial officer can make an informed decision in regards to purchasing the item.

VENDORS

There are many different ways to find equipment vendors, and it is important to shop around, especially when making capital equipment purchases. Some vendors may offer discounts for multiple sales, a large scale, or to specific organizations. Discounts may also be offered to organizations that frequently buy from a specific vendor.

When shopping for equipment, it is often helpful to examine and use the equipment in person as well as read the specifications. Therefore, it is advisable to visit local supplies and trade shows to view sample items. Before buying, however, check the catalogs and websites of other vendors. When buying, compare price against specifications and warranty. Some vendors will add extended warranties to their product for an additional cost.

EQUIPMENT SPECIFICATIONS

Information compiled for an equipment specification should include the following:

- Name
- Dimensions
- Capacity
- Energy and/or power needs
- Warranty
- Delivery requirements
- Approval/Certifications needed
- Training Requirements
- Interior and exterior construction materials
- Additional features and/or accessories needed
- Compatibility with available space, kitchen design, and other equipment
- Ability to fulfill the current and projected needs of the organization

PREVENTATIVE MAINTENANCE

Preventative maintenance is a schedule of cleaning, fixing, and tuning-up equipment to increase its life. It is important that all equipment, especially capital equipment undergo routine preventative maintenance and inspections to ensure the item is operating properly and safely. Though preventative maintenance may seem to be a hassle, it prevents serious inconvenience in the long-term. Preventative maintenance increases the life of a product, reduces costs associated with fixing and replacing the item, ensures employee safety, and maximizes the organization's resources. The unanticipated failure of equipment may lead to more labor costs as the organization attempts to purchase additional equipment.

ORGANIZATIONS THAT REVIEW AND APPROVE FOOD SERVICE EQUIPMENT

There are four nationally recognized organizations that review, approve, and certify food service equipment. Those organizations are the National Sanitation Foundation (NSF), Underwriters Laboratories (UL), American Gas Association (AGA), and International Standards Organization (ISO). NSF, UL, and AGA certify products. NSF and UL designate approval via a seal. UL approves electrical appliances. AGA grants a certification for gas appliances that meet their safety standards. Unlike the others, ISO certifies a manufacturer, not the individual products. Buying products that have met the certification standards of one or more of the above organizations ensures that a quality, inspected item is purchased.

COMMON SAFETY FEATURES

It is important that food service equipment be designed with safety in mind. Some equipment may have safety features built in whereas others may be fitted with extraneous parts and/or an

75

employee may wear protective garments to ensure safety. Some standard safety equipment features include:

- Blade guards on mixers and food slicers
- Automatic shutoff for electronic equipment
- Exhaust hoods and/or other escape
- Hot service indicators
- Protective gloves, potholders, handles, etc.
- Cord storage

FOOD TYPES

ORGANIC FOODS

Recent years have seen a shift in food production in which growers are producing and marketing "organic" foods. Organic foods are those that are grown without the use of pesticides, synthesized fertilizers, and without exposure to human waste or sewage. Animal products that are certified organic are not typically injected with growth hormone or antibiotics. Additionally, many of the animals are raised on organic feed and do not have any genetic modifications.

In the United States, the United States Department of Agriculture has adopted the National Organic Program, which certifies organic foods based upon the standards set forth by that program.

SEAFOOD

As with other types of food, it is important that seafood, including fish and shellfish be purchased from an approved, regulated vendor. Buying outside of regulated vendors may put customers at risk of contamination and illness and, therefore, may jeopardize the health and reputation of an organization. Seafood, like other foods, is regulated by the United States Food and Drug Administration. The FDA has paired with other nation's food safety agencies to evaluate and approve certain shellfish vendors. Those vendor's names are included on the Interstate Certified Shellfish Shippers List. Buyers may purchase shellfish (edible pieces of oysters, clams, mussels, and scallops) with confidence from these vendors. Many states also have regulations governing seafood distribution with respective vendor lists. These may also serve as a resource for safe seafood purchase.

According to the United States Food and Drug Administration (US FDA), the following characteristics generally indicate seafood freshness:

- Mild smell, not overly fishy or ammonia-like.
- Clear, slightly bulging eyes, not sunken or cloudy.
- Skin that is firm and shiny.
- Bright red gills, free from slime.
- Springy flesh.
- Fillets that are free from discoloration (brown, yellow, or green) do not appear mushy, dry, or dark.

When buying frozen fish, be sure that the package is fully sealed and free from holes and sits lower in the store's freezer. Additionally, if the fish is visible through the package, avoid buying fish that has a dry appearance and/or is covered with frost or ice.

FOOD STORAGE
GENERAL FOOD STORAGE GUIDELINES

Food must not only be stored at proper temperatures, but in an orderly fashion that prevents contamination of food by humans, other foods, and pests. Therefore, the following guidelines apply to food storage:

- Store food on shelves that are at least 6" from the ground.
- Store food away from walls and ceilings.
- Store food in containers that protect products from contamination or infestation.
- Store food in such a way to avoid cross-contamination:
- Sort and store meat and poultry products by type.
- Store pre-cooked and ready-to-eat foods above raw meats, poultry, seafood, etc., to avoid contamination from leaking juices.
- Store food away from chemicals, cleansers, leaks, and any other source of contamination.
- Do not store food in restrooms, changing areas, stairwells, or any other area that may be contaminated by human waste and germs.
- Store food in a well-ventilated, cool, dry area.

STORAGE TEMPERATURES

Appropriate storage temperatures are as follows:

$$Freezer = 0°F, maximum$$
$$Deep\ Chill = 26°F - 32°F$$
$$Refrigerator = 41°F, maximum$$
$$Dry\ Storage = 50°F - 70°F$$

It is important that foods be stored at (or in the case of freezer and refrigerator storage, below) their respective storage temperatures to maintain the integrity of the product. Storing food above the designated temperature introduces the risk of spoilage and contamination. It is particularly dangerous to allow food needing refrigeration to sit at a temperature between 40°F-140°F, as it is in this range that it is easiest for bacteria to grow and multiply

MEAT PRODUCTS

It is important to properly store all food products to ensure that the items do not become susceptible to foodborne pathogens that may cause illness to clients. Additionally, taste and texture of foods deteriorate with the item's shelf-life. If stored at the correct temperatures, which is 0°F for frozen meats and at or below 41°F for refrigerated foods, beef may be stored in the freezer for approximately 6-12 months. Refrigerated beef should be used within 3-6 days of purchase. Ground beef should only be stored for 3-4 months in the freezer and up to 2 days in the refrigerator. If, upon thawing, evidence of freezer burn, discoloration, or odor is present, it is best to dispose of the beef entirely.

POULTRY AND EGG PRODUCTS

It is important to properly store all food products to ensure that the items do not become susceptible to foodborne pathogens that may cause illness to clients. Additionally, taste and texture of foods deteriorate with the item's shelf-life. Poultry and egg products should be refrigerated at a temperature no greater than 41°F and should be frozen at or below 0°F. Poultry has a shelf-life of approximately 6 months when stored in a freezer but should be used within a couple of days if refrigerated. Eggs and egg products shelf-life differ, based on the type of product. Generally speaking, fresh eggs should be used within 1-2 weeks of purchase. For egg products that are packed or in a carton, check the use by label on the carton for guidance.

SEAFOOD PRODUCTS

It is important to properly store all food products to ensure that the items do not become susceptible to foodborne pathogens that may cause illness to clients. Additionally, taste and texture of foods deteriorate with the item's shelf-life. Seafood products may last as long as 4 months when properly stored in a freezer at a temperature no higher than 0°F. If refrigerated, at a temperature at or below 41°F, seafood products are safe to prepare up to two days after the date of purchase. Do not prepare seafood that appears discolored, freezer-burned, or has a particularly fishy odor. Seafood in that condition should be disposed of immediately.

DAIRY PRODUCTS

It is important to properly store all food products to ensure that the items do not become susceptible to foodborne pathogens that may cause illness to clients. Additionally, taste and texture of foods deteriorate with the item's shelf-life. Dairy products have a wide range of shelf-lives depending upon whether the item is pasteurized, processed, and the type of product. Always use the expiration date on the carton or packaging as a guide for using and disposing dairy products. Generally speaking, dairy products should be stored at a maximum temperature of 41°F in the refrigerator and a maximum temperature of 0°F in the freezer. Some dairy products packaged in UHT packaging may be stored at room temperature, if the package remains unopened.

SHELF-LIFE
BASIC STAPLES

Every food product has a shelf-life. Taste and texture of foods deteriorate with time, and many foods may spoil, leading to a health hazard for consumers. Look to the food packaging for specific dates regarding shelf-life. Below are some general guidelines in regards to shelf life:

- Baking powder: 18 months
- Baking soda: 2 years
- Chocolate: 18 months
- Coffee can, unopened: 2 years
- Corn Syrup: 3 years
- Cornstarch: 18 months
- Flour: 6-8 months
- Honey: 12 months
- Rice, white: 2 years
- Rice, brown: 6-12 months
- Shortening: 8 months
- Sugar, granulated: 2 years
- Sugar, brown: 4 months
- Vinegar, unopened: 2 years

TERMS

Many food products are labeled with a date. It is important to understand the definition of these terms so that food is properly stored, used, and disposed of when necessary. The terms are defined below.

"Sell by date": The last date by which a product should be sold from the retailer. These dates allow consumers a period of a few days past the designated date to use the product.

"Expiration date": The last day that a food product should be consumed or used for cooking. It is prudent to dispose of food that has passed its expiration date.

"Use by date": The date product may start losing its freshness.

"Packed on date": The day on which a food was canned, packaged, and/or processed.

FIFO

FIFO is the acronym for "First In, First Out." The "first in, first out" principle is a guideline for using, moving, and handling food. When an organization receives a delivery of food, the older products should be rotated to the front of the shelf, and the new products placed behind the older products. When the food stores are rotated in this manner, it ensures that food is used in the order it is received, thus minimizing food waste. Even with proper rotation, it is important that food dates always be checked prior to using and/or serving food products to ensure that the food is still safe for consumption.

TTI Strips

Time/temperature indicator (TTI) strips are also known as shelf-life indicators. These strips change color to indicate whether a product is still considered fresh or safe. The indicator is programmed to change when a product reaches its expiration date or if it has been stored incorrectly, thus resulting in the possibility of spoilage. The TTI strip should be examined when receiving goods and any products with a changed strip should be rejected and disposed of properly. Never serve or use products whose indicator strips have changed color, as it poses unnecessary risk to consumers.

PACKAGING AND SHIPPING
PACKAGING PROCESSES

Ultra-pasteurization is a food processing option that uses extremely high heat, of at least 280°F, for a short period of time, generally a matter of seconds, to kill microorganisms and harmful bacteria in food. This process is effective in prolonging the shelf-life of foods; however, it does not eliminate the need for refrigeration. Some ultra-pasteurized foods are also packaged in ultra-high temperature (UHT) packaging. UHT packaging is aseptic. As a result, foods that are processed through ultra-pasteurization and ultra-high temperature packaging do not ultimately require refrigeration and are considered stable for shelf storage.

RECEIVING A FOOD SHIPMENT

It is important to assign shipment receiving to a trained employee, as the incoming food must be checked for quality assurance purposes. Food that does not meet the quality and safety standards of an organization should not be accepted from the vendor, and a refund should be immediately requested. The following is a list of quality indicators that should be checked during receipt of a shipment:

- Temperature of potentially hazardous foods (PHF/TCS).
- Packaging: Reject products with defective, suspect, or tampered packaging.
- Inspection stamps and dates.
- Food expiration and/or use-by dates.
- Quality of food, to include color, texture, and odor.

FOOD VENDOR SELECTION

Food vendors abound, and it is, therefore, important to carefully select vendors from which to order an organization's food supplies. A vendor must be reliable in all regards, including food quality and safety, prompt and courteous delivery, reasonable prices, etc. Below are some things to consider when selecting a food vendor:

- Quality of vendor's products and service.
- Willingness to schedule convenient deliveries for organization.
- Willingness to have all deliveries inspected.
- Willingness to refund monies for food rejected at delivery.
- Quality of vendor's equipment, to include storage facility/warehouse, delivery trucks, refrigerator/freezer equipment.
- Vendor's reputation and record of service.
- Follows a HACCP process.
- Subjects itself to inspection and willing to present inspection findings to customers.

Food Production, Distribution, and Service

MEASUREMENT EQUIVALENTS

Common cooking volume, weight, and fluid measurement equivalent are as follows:

$$3 \text{ teaspoons} = 1 \text{ tablespoon}$$
$$16 \text{ tablespoons} = 1 \text{ cup}$$
$$8 \text{ ounces} = 1 \text{ cup}$$
$$2 \text{ cups} = 1 \text{ pint}$$
$$2 \text{ pints} = 1 \text{ quart}$$
$$4 \text{ quarts} = 1 \text{ gallon}$$
$$8 \text{ quarts} = 2 \text{ gallons} = 1 \text{ peck}$$
$$8 \text{ gallons} = 4 \text{ pecks} = 1 \text{ bushel}$$
$$16 \text{ ounces} = 1 \text{ pound}$$

TYPES OF SERVICE SYSTEMS

TRAY-LINE SERVICE SYSTEM

A tray-line system is a streamlined method of preparing trays for clients. This system operates in an assembly-line fashion in which trays are passed (either manually or by conveyor belt) from one food service worker to another. In the instances where clients are given menu options, foods are most often grouped according to where they fall on the menu. As the trays are passed, food service workers prepare trays using the selected menu items for each individual. It is important that tray-line employees ensure that menu selections match the finished tray and that trays are handled quickly and efficiently. Employee distractions may result in a health risk to clients as delayed delivery of food compromises the temperature of the prepared items.

CONTROLLING TEMPERATURE: There are many tools and procedures available to ensure proper temperature control of food originating at a tray-line. For example, an institution may choose to deliver food on an insulated tray or utilizing dinnerware that contains warming plates. Additionally, many tray transporters have temperature controlling properties, whether those consist of insulation or continuous heat. Finally, quick tray assembly and prompt delivery of the food is paramount. Not only does quick delivery promote correct temperature at delivery but it also enhances the attractiveness of the plate, as foods are not allowed the opportunity to "wilt."

<u>**EFFICIENCY STUDY**</u>: A tray-line efficiency study is a method of evaluating the effectiveness, quickness, and organization of a tray-line. A study can be carried out via a variety of methods. One such method is to calculate the number of trays per minute leaving the tray-line. Another method is to intercept a sample of the trays between assembly and delivery and to calculate the rate of accuracy of prepared trays compared to selected menu items. Additionally, randomly testing trays between assembly and delivery for proper food temperature is another method of determining tray-line efficiency. A tray-line efficiency study is important in that it allows a dietary manager to see a greater picture of what is happening on the tray-line. If food is being served cold, perhaps the assembly is taking too long. If a menu item is not being properly served, there may be an issue with a tray-line employee. Furthermore, tray-line efficiency studies may be helpful in justifying additional hires of food service employees.

<u>**TRAYS PER MINUTE CALCULATION**</u>: A trays per minute calculation is most often included in a tray-line efficiency study. To calculate trays per minute, one must first record the amount of time it takes to assemble trays. Do this by timing from the beginning of tray assembly until the last tray leaves the tray-line. Measure the time in minutes. Next, count the number of trays that left the line during the recorded time. Now, divide the number of trays assembled by the number of recorded minutes. So, if a tray-line was operating for thirty minutes and ninety trays were assembled, one would calculate the trays per minute by using the following equation:

(Trays assembled) / (Minutes of assembly) = Trays per minute

(90 trays) / (30 minutes) = 3 trays per minute

<u>**TRAY-LINE ACCURACY**</u>: Tray-line accuracy is used to estimate the number of errors occurring during tray-line assembly. Accuracy rates are important determinants of tray-line efficiency. Fewer tray errors mean greater efficiency. To calculate tray-line accuracy, select a random sampling of trays. A greater sample size will produce more accurate data; however, one should be mindful of time when performing a tray-line accuracy survey. Delaying trays for the sake of the study is unacceptable. Using the tray tickets, count the total number of items for each tray, and add those tray totals together. Next, compare the tray ticket to the actual tray. Count the number of errors. Errors could include missing items, serving an item incorrectly, and/or inclusion of unordered items. Then, divide the total number of errors by the total number of ordered tray-line items. The product will equal the percent error. The smaller the error, the greater the tray-line accuracy. An example follows:

> Tray 1 (T1): 10 items, 1 error; T2: 12 items, 0 errors; T3: 11 items, 2 errors; T4: 12 items, 3 errors. Total number of errors: 6
> Total number of items: 45   Percent error: [(6 errors)/ (45 items)] x 100 = 13%
> Thus, the tray is accurate 87% of the time.

BUFFET

This type of service is one in which all menu items are displayed buffet style, usually on temperature regulated tables conducive to self-service. Clients are able to browse the items and select the items that they would like to consume. Generally, buffets include a wide-range of menu options. Foods are typically grouped according to temperature and compatibility. Additionally, buffets give clients the freedom to choose their own portion sizes.

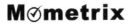

FAMILY-STYLE

Family-style dinner service is such that customers sitting at a table pass serving dishes to one another. Each person is able to choose the food he/she is interested in as well as the portion. Menu options are limited to a specific meal.

CAFETERIA SERVICE

Cafeteria service is a method of food service in which customers may select from a wide variety of items to assemble an individual meal. There are a various types of cafeteria models. Some arrangements promote self-service while others require a food service worker to serve the client. Some cafeterias are arranged such that a client must follow a line and select foods as he/she moves along. Conversely, many cafeterias have adopted a "scramble system" in which customers may float from station to station to choose menu items. The advantage of this system is that a client does not have to wait in line unnecessarily, and therefore, scramble systems generally promote faster food service.

WAIT VS. SELF-SERVICE

Wait-service refers to the type of food service wherein wait staff brings prepared plates to the tables and present the plates to clients. Depending upon the size of the staff and institutional procedures, the roles and responsibilities of wait staff vary. This type of service is labor intensive and is not often utilized at institutions because of the high labor costs. On the other hand, self-service is when a client serves him/herself. This method is effective in minimizing costs as food service staff may be kept at a minimum. It does, however, promote the greatest freedom of dietary choice, which can undermine the purpose of therapeutic diets.

KITCHEN EQUIPMENT

UTENSIL STORAGE

It is important to store all clean and sanitized dinnerware in a manner that prevents contamination. Therefore, utensils stored in a cylindrical container should be placed with the handles facing upwards. Additionally, cups, bowls, and other concave dinnerware should be stored face down on clean, dry, dust-free shelves or racks. All dinnerware should be kept on clean, dry, flat, dust-free surfaces. Moreover, dinnerware should be stored off the floor and in a manner that prevents contamination from food, chemical, and other spills. Food service employees should be careful to follow proper hand washing procedure when stacking items for storage and/or accessing dinnerware to prepare a plate.

CUTTING BOARDS

Wooden cutting boards are not generally recommended for food preparation, and in fact, this type of cutting board is often prohibited. Cutting boards are highly susceptible to bacteria growth and transferring foodborne pathogens as they come in contact in with a variety of foods and surfaces. For this reason, it is imperative to use cutting boards that are scratch resistant, usually of specific acrylic or rubber materials. If a cutting board shows evidence of scratching or scoring, it should immediately be replaced. Moreover, proper cleaning and sanitizing methods must be used for cutting boards to eliminate any foodborne pathogens lingering on the surface of the equipment. It is advisable to designate cutting boards for use with only one type of food, meat, vegetables, chicken, etc., to further eliminate cross-contamination.

KITCHEN EQUIPMENT LAYOUT

Food service areas should be designed in a manner that promotes a fast, effective flow of traffic while minimizing the need for workers to access various areas of a kitchen. Moreover, a kitchen

82

should be laid out in such a manner that energy and light sources are effectively utilized without being overburdened. Therefore, equipment should be grouped according to function so that preparation areas are in one location, refrigerators and freezers are adjacent to one another, and grills, fryers, and ovens are in convenient proximity to one another. Food preparation areas should be as far from chemical storage and cleaning areas as possible. Service areas should be designed such that food servers do not have to pass through the cooking area. Traffic areas should be wide enough to adequately handle the number of people necessary for the kitchen demand.

Sanitation, Safety, Equipment, and Facilities

FOOD SAFETY
CRITICAL CONTROL POINT (CCP)

A critical control point is a limit set in order to ensure food safety. At this limit, controls can be applied such that food hazards are eliminated and/or are reduced to a level within the acceptable parameters. The most common application of critical control points is in cooking, where temperatures are assigned to determine safety of various foods. Those measures, when taken at the thickest part of a meat are as follows:

- 135° -- Cooked fruits, vegetables, and any commercially processed food that will be held for an extended period before being consumed.
- 145° -- Roasts, steaks, chops, fish, eggs.
- 155° -- Ground meats or fish, injected meats, eggs that will not be immediately consumed.
- 165° -- Poultry, stuffing, stuffed items (including meats, fish, pasta, and poultry), any food that was allowed to cool and/or was refrigerated and that will be reheated from a temperature below 135°.

**Note: Temperatures must be sustained for varying amounts of time, usually ranging from 4-15 seconds.

Seven principles of Hazard Analysis Critical Control Point (HACCP)

- *Principle 1:* Conduct a hazard analysis in which any food safety hazard, such as those presented by chemical, biological or physical composition and/or properties is determined.
- *Principle 2:* Determine critical control points by setting limits that serve to eliminate and/or reduce any potential food risk.
- *Principle 3:* Develop preventative measures, to include critical limits, for each critical control point.
- *Principle 4:* Institute critical control point monitoring procedures. These monitoring procedures and the frequency with which they are carried out must be listed in the HACCP plan.
- *Principle 5:* Develop corrective actions that will rectify any situation in which the monitoring procedures show that critical limits have not been reached.
- *Principle 6:* Verify that all procedures as well as the HACCP system are correctly working.
- *Principle 7:* Institute an efficient data system to document and maintain HACCP system records.

Hazard Analysis Critical Control Point records should include the following information:

- An analysis summary which outlines and justifies the hazards and control points.
- The HACCP plan, including information about the team and responsibilities of each individual, description of food and services to the consumer, a flow diagram of the process, and a plan summary. The plan summary should incorporate each of the seven principles (critical control points, critical limits, applicable hazards, monitoring, corrective actions, verification, and records log).
- Supporting documentation.
- Information logged during the implementation of the plan.

SAFE TEMPERATURES

It is important that food shipments/purchases be tested for proper temperature before signing in receipt of the goods. Food delivered at temperatures above that at which they should be stored is susceptible to spoilage. In the case of such a delivery, the food from that delivery should be thrown out. Poultry, seafood, meat, and egg products should all be received at or below 41°F if refrigerated and below 0°F if frozen. Dairy products should be received at a temperature between 6°F and 10°F, if frozen. Otherwise, dairy products should be refrigerated below 41°F.

WHEN FOOD PACKAGING COMPROMISES MAY PRESENT A HEALTH RISK

The quality of packaged food may be compromised when the packaging is disturbed, torn, dented, or defective in anyway. When receiving food purchases, it is important to check all packaging for flaws and disturbance. Be particularly vigilant of packages that show evidence of dents, rust, tears, leaks, or other damage and/or tampering. These products should be rejected at delivery or disposed of if the damage occurs between delivery and use. Additionally, eggs that are delivered with cracked or discolored shells should also be discarded. It is never prudent to prepare meals using food from damaged containers.

FOODBORNE ILLNESSES

Foodborne illness is any type of disease or pathogen that is transmitted by food or food products. Foodborne illness most often manifests with "flu-like" symptoms, to include diarrhea, vomiting, fever, headache, chills, and others, though it may take on other symptoms. In severe cases, foodborne illness may lead to death. These types of illnesses are not transferable from one person to another, as the cause of the illness is linked to consumed food. When two or more people contract a foodborne illness from the same food, and chemical analyses confirm that the food was the culprit of the illness, a foodborne illness "outbreak" is declared.

TYPES OF HAZARDS THAT MAY LEAD TO FOODBORNE ILLNESS

Foodborne illness is caused by a variety of contaminating factors. Those factors are divided into three broad categories: biological pathogens, chemical hazards, and physical contaminants. Biological pathogens include: bacteria (including e coli), viruses, parasites, natural toxins, fungi, and prions. Chemical hazards include contamination by cleaning supplies, pesticides sprayed on crops, and materials used during production, manufacturing, and packaging. Physical contaminants include dirt, body/animal hair, bone, shards of plastic, metal, glass, wood, rocks and other materials.

FATAL FOODBORNE ILLNESSES

Foodborne illnesses may, in fact, be fatal if not properly detected or treated. While most foodborne illness will pass within a matter of hours or days, some illness can be so severely dehydrating and/or may attack one's immune system in such a way that they are fatal.

Typical symptoms of foodborne illness include nausea, vomiting, diarrhea, muscle pain, fever, abdominal pain, difficulties swallowing, breathing, or speaking, headache, chills, cramping, and dehydration. Illness onset may be anywhere from one hour to a matter of days, depending upon the type of pathogen. All foodborne illnesses should be reported.

BACTERIAL PATHOGENS

STAPHYLOCOCCUS AUREUS

S. aureus is a commonly occurring bacterium that lives in nasal passages and in cuts on the skin. Infection with the toxin can be avoided when proper food handling practices are observed. Foods should be refrigerated promptly and at the proper temperature. Observe good hand-washing practices, and keep cuts and abrasions bandaged. S. aureus produces toxins when contaminated foods are left at room temperature for prolonged periods. Common culprits include protein-rich foods such as meats, poultry, eggs, mayonnaise-based salads, and cream filled pastry products. Symptoms mimic the flu, but are rarely fatal, and can include diarrhea, vomiting, and abdominal cramps. The illness comes on quickly, within a few hours after eating, and can last 24-48 hours.

SALMONELLA

A variety of Salmonella bacteria cause thousands of cases in the U.S. each year. Illness comes from consuming the live bacteria, which are toxic. The bacteria thrive in animal and human feces and enter the food chain through dirty cutting boards, infected water, contaminated meat, broken or cracked eggs, or actual bits of feces in foodstuffs. The symptoms are similar to those of Staphylococcus aureus, but take longer to develop, up to 72 hours. Symptoms are flu-like and include nausea and vomiting, headache, diarrhea, and abdominal cramps. Salmonella infection can be avoided by refrigerating eggs, meat, and poultry products at the proper temperatures. Care should be taken to sanitize food preparation surfaces after contact with raw meats or eggs to avoid cross-contamination. Consuming undercooked eggs, meat and poultry puts one at risk for Salmonella, but thorough cooking kills the bacteria.

CLOSTRIDIUM BOTULINUM

C. botulinum is a rare but deadly microbe commonly occurring in the soil and probably in most foodstuffs. However, the bacteria thrive in an anaerobic environment, and botulism cases in the U.S. are rare. Common sources of botulism poisoning include canned products, especially home-canned products with low acidity, such as meat, corn, beans, and asparagus. Commercially canned products can harbor the toxin as well, and cans should be inspected for bulges, rust, or milky fluid. Any canned foods bearing signs of spoilage should be discarded, as one bite-sized portion can harbor enough toxins to be fatal. Symptoms include vomiting, dizziness, and respiratory failure. Treatment is possible with a quick diagnosis, but recovery may take weeks. Botulism poisoning can also occur in infants under the age of one year who ingest honey, as their stomach acidity is not strong enough to kill the spores sometimes found in honey. Following proper home-canning procedures advocated by the USDA can reduce the risk of this rare foodborne illness.

LISTERIA MONOCYTOGENES

The source of infection with L. monocytogenes can be difficult to pinpoint, as the onset of symptoms may not occur until several days or even a few weeks after ingesting the contaminated food. Symptoms may include fever, headache, or vomiting, but susceptible individuals such as pregnant women, infants, and those with suppressed immune function may suffer more severe symptoms or even death. The bacteria are much more resilient than other foodborne pathogens and can resist heat, temperatures below 40 degrees, and acidity. Common sources include unpasteurized dairy products, such as semi-soft cheeses like brie. Deli meats and hot dogs have also been implicated, and pregnant women are advised to heat these products to 160 degrees and steaming before

85

consumption. Individuals at high risk should avoid consuming semi-soft cheeses and other unpasteurized dairy products or products made with raw milk.

CANNED GOODS

There are many types of bacteria and these bacteria grow under a variety of conditions. For example, aerobic bacteria must have exposure to oxygen to live and grow whereas anaerobic bacteria do not have that need. Some bacteria can grow with or without oxygen; those types are called facultative. Therefore, it is possible for bacteria to grow, even in canned goods or from the center of foods. The danger of bacterial growth and/or bacteria-released toxins is much higher when food packaging is damaged; therefore, it is important to reject all items with packaging defects.

CONDITIONS UNDER WHICH BACTERIA ARE LIKELY TO GROW

Bacteria are microorganisms, and as such, it requires certain conditions to grow. Those conditions include:

- Appropriate temperature. The typical danger zone for bacterial growth is between 41°F - 135°F.
- Presence of oxygen, depending upon the type of bacteria.
- Time exposure. It is best not to serve food that has been in the "danger zone" for an extended period of time (between 2-4 hours).
- Moisture.
- pH of food; bacteria is more likely to grow in slightly acidic conditions.
- Nutrient composition.

COMMON TYPES OF BACTERIAL PATHOGENS

There are many types of foodborne bacterial pathogens. Some of the most commonly encountered pathogens include:

- Aeromonas hydrophilia
- Bacillus cereus
- Campylobacter jejuni
- Clostridium botulinum
- Clostridium perfringens
- Listeria monocytogenes
- Salmonella enteritidis
- Shiga Toxin-Producing Escherichia coli
- Shigella
- Staphylococcus aureus
- Vibrio cholerae
- Vibrio parahaemolyticus
- Yersinia enterocolitica

FOODBORNE VIRUSES

Viruses that are contracted from the consumption of food are often classified as gastroenteritis viruses. These viruses most often cause symptoms such as nausea, vomiting, diarrhea, and abdominal cramping. Foodborne viruses are generally spread from person-to-person, in that an infected food service worker may contaminate foods later consumed by a customer. Additionally, certain foods, namely seafood, can carry viruses. While viruses are life forms, they do not grow on or in foods. Some of the most common foodborne viruses include: Hepatitis A and E, Norovirus, and Rotavirus.

FOODBORNE PARASITES

Parasites are organisms that live and feed off of a "host," which is another living organism. Foodborne parasites include worms, insects, and protozoa. Parasites are most commonly found in meat and seafood, though they may be present on fruits and vegetables as well as in milk and water. Common symptoms of parasites include muscle pain, abdominal cramping, fever, diarrhea, bloating, weight loss, and symptoms of malnourishment as the body is not given the opportunity to absorb important vitamins, minerals, and nutrients.

Commonly identified foodborne parasites include:

- Acanthamoeba
- Anisakis
- Ascaris lumbricoides
- Cryptosporidium parvum
- Cyclospora cayetanensis
- Diphyllobothrium
- Entamoeba histolytica
- Giardia lamblia
- Nanophyetus
- Trichinella spiralis
- Trichuris trichiura

FOODBORNE FUNGI

Fungus is most often present in foods in the forms of mold or yeast. Sometimes, therefore, fungus is helpful in producing foods, such as the production of yeast-breads and cheeses (mold). However, these types of fungi may also be hazardous, in that they can release toxins called mycotoxins. The types of mycotoxins that commonly appear in food include: aflatoxins, deoxynivalenol, fumonisin, nivalenol, ochratoxin A, and zearalenone. Mycotoxins may lead to serious neurological problems, and several mycotoxins are suspected to be carcinogens. Mold typically appears as a dark greenish-black, fuzzy growth on the surface of food. Most fungi, mold spores in particular, need three things to grow: moisture, time, and some sort of nutrient, generally of organic material. Yeast may spoil food through a process of fermentation, which may be detected by food discoloration or an alcohol-like odor.

SAFELY CONSUMED MOLD

Many foods may be safely consumed even if mold is present on the product. It is important, however, to cut away the moldy part of the food as well as a one-inch section of the food surrounding the mold. Mold may be removed from the following items, which can later be safely served: Apples, bell peppers, broccoli, brussel sprouts, cabbage, cauliflower, firm cheeses (i.e., Swiss, cheddar), garlic, onions, pears, potatoes, turnips, winter squash, and zucchini. Cheeses that are intentionally moldy, such as blue, gorgonzola, and stilton varieties may be consumed without cutting out the visible mold.

PRIONS

Prions are pathogens that are entirely comprised of damaged or mutated proteins. These pathogens attack the neurological system of animals and humans. The neurodegenesis is untreatable and fatal. Prions are responsible for "mad-cow disease," bovine spongiform encephalopathy. Prions are responsible for Creutzfeldt-Jakob disease, Gerstmann-Strauussler-Scheinker syndrome, fatal familial insomnia, sporadic fatal insomnia, Kuru, and Alpers syndrome. Prions are only infectious when consumed as part of an animal source.

Prion infection is highly unlikely, though risk does exist. The greatest risk of infection by prions occurs when bovine neural tissue (brain, spinal cord, nerves) and/or parts of the small intestines are consumed.

NATURAL TOXINS

Toxins naturally occur in some plants and animals. Natural toxins are most commonly found in seafood and mushrooms. Often times, toxins in seafood develop after the sea animal eats from algae. Naturally occurring toxins may also be present in red beans and honey. Symptoms resulting from illness caused by natural toxins are primarily neurological though it is not uncommon to experience gastrointestinal symptoms such as vomiting, diarrhea, and abdominal cramping. Some natural toxins also affect the human cardiovascular system. The most effective way to avoid naturally occurring toxins is to buy seafood and mushrooms from reliable, approved, and inspected sources.

HIGHLY SUSCEPTIBLE POPULATIONS

Highly susceptible populations are those in which there is a greater risk of contracting an illness or experiencing the illness and its symptoms more severely than in normal populations. Children, the elderly, pregnant women, and individuals with suppressed immune system functioning are all considered highly susceptible populations. These populations are not only more likely to experience more severe symptoms of foodborne illness but the peripheral effects, such as malabsorption of nutrients and dehydration are more drastic, and therefore, more difficult to recover from than in a healthy adult. Accordingly, the Food and Drug Administration (FDA) stipulates that greater care must be taken when serving these populations in order to protect them from foodborne illness.

The FDA Food Code mandates that eggs, juices, and fresh seed sprouts must be handled with additional care. The FDA Food Code prohibits serving eggs that are not fully cooked to highly susceptible populations. This regulation applies to meringues, soufflés, soft-cooked eggs, and raw eggs among others. Additionally, it is highly recommended that treated egg products or pasteurized eggs be used for any recipe in which more than one egg is called for. Juices must also be processed or pasteurized before serving to highly susceptible populations. Fresh seed sprouts and raw meats are strictly prohibited by the Food Code for service to these populations.

CROSS-CONTAMINATION

Cross-contamination is the transfer of pathogens from any item to food during the production, preparation, and service of food items. Cross-contamination is a major cause of foodborne illness and should be avoided. Food can easily be contaminated by coming in contact with other foods, contaminated equipment, or an individual who is carrying a pathogen. Cross-contamination often occurs when equipment is not properly cleaned between uses and/or the food service worker does not follow correct hand washing and handling procedure. Additionally, cross-contamination is likely to occur when unwashed produce or raw meats come in contact with clean, ready to eat foods.

Cross-contamination may be prevented by following some simple guidelines. Those include:

- Thoroughly wash hands between handling food, after using the restroom and/or performing any personal grooming.
- Store cooked and raw foods separate from one another. Never store raw foods above cooked foods, to avoid spillage of juices.
- Do not use the same cutting board and knife to cut cooked foods as was used for raw foods.
- Thoroughly wash and sanitize all utensils and equipment that comes in contact with food.
- Keep washed and unwashed foods away from one another.

MANAGING WASTE TO AVOID CROSS-CONTAMINATION OF FOODS

As with all other aspects of food service, waste should be carefully and deliberately managed to avoid contamination of foods. Waste receptacles should be regularly cleaned, sanitized and should be fitted with tight lids. The receptacles should be free from defects, which may allow leaking or seepage of discarded materials. Trash should regularly be removed from the food service area to an outdoor dumpster. Moreover, trash receptacles should be placed in the farthest possible location from food preparation areas. Outdoor dumpsters should also be fitted with tightly fitted lids, and the area surrounding the dumpsters should be maintained for cleanliness. It is also advisable to install lighting around the dumpster to ensure employee safety.

PROPER THAWING TECHNIQUES

Food should never be thawed on a kitchen counter. Doing so allows the food to sit in the "hazard" zone for a lengthy amount of time, putting the item at risk for bacterial growth and foodborne pathogens. Rather, food should be thawed in the refrigerator, at a temperature no greater than 41°F. Food may also be thawed by placing it in an airtight, watertight plastic bag, and submerged in cold water. The water should remain running or should, at least, be changed every 20 minutes. In some cases, food may be thawed in the oven during cooking. Generally, frozen foods will take at least 1.5 times as long as those already thawed to cook. Finally, food may be thawed completely in a microwave. Use this method only if the food will be cooked entirely immediately after thawing.

MONITORING FOOD TEMPERATURE

It is important to know how to measure food temperatures accurately, as a food thermometer may be the most effective tool in warning that food may be subject to foodborne illness. To correctly measure food temperature, it is important to use a food thermometer. Insert the thermometer into the center and/or thickest part of the food item, being careful to avoid touching bone, fat, or any part of the pan. In the case of frozen items, a thermometer may be inserted between frozen packages of food. Regardless of whether the temperature of hot or cold foods is being measured, it is important to leave the thermometer in place for several seconds to ensure an accurate reading. Finally, the thermometer must be thoroughly washed and sanitized between uses.

DEVICES AVAILABLE TO MEASURE THE TEMPERATURE OF FOODS

It is important that foods be heated to an appropriate endpoint temperature. To ensure that foods reach the endpoint temperature, one should measure the internal temperature of a food with a food thermometer. Typically, a bi-metallic stem thermometer is used to measure the internal temperature of larger portions of food. These thermometers generally require that a fairly large surface area, close to 3" of the probe be in contact with the interior portion of the food being measured. When a large measuring surface area is not available, it is important to use a smaller-diameter probe, such as a thermistor or thermocouple thermometer.

RETAINING THE TEMPERATURE OF HOT FOODS

Hot foods must be maintained at a temperature of at least 135ºF (140 ºF, according to some sources). Food may be kept at this temperature by using warming plates, steaming tables, and other specialized equipment. When holding and transporting food, it is important that foods maintain a healthy and safe temperature. Thus, it is imperative that temperature be measured frequently, at least every two hours. If the temperature falls below a safe measurement, the food should be immediately reheated or discarded. In the case of buffet or tray line service, it is also recommended that an entire pan of food act as a refill. In other words, fresh, hot food should not be poured onto food that has been sitting.

HOLDING COLD FOODS

As with hot holding, cold holding is regulated by the food temperature. Foods should stay at or below a temperature of 41 ºF, to maintain the safety and integrity of the food. Food may be transported in refrigerator units or may be placed in ice baths, except when packaging may allow water or ice to come into direct contact with the food. Generally speaking, unpackaged foods may not come into contact with undrained ice. Again, it is imperative that temperatures be regularly monitored and logged to ensure the safety of foods. During food service, utensils may be in contact with the food, however, between uses, the utensils should be stored in water that is at least 135 ºF.

LEFTOVERS

If leftover food is handled correctly, it may be served again. Follow these tips for storing, reheating, and serving leftovers:

- Discard food that has been at room temperature for more than two hours.
- Quick-chill or separate food into small containers to cool before placing in the refrigerator.
- Refrigerate leftovers immediately (or once cooled by quick-chilling/dividing into smaller containers).
- Reheat leftovers to at least 165°F before serving.
- Do not reheat leftovers more than once. Discard remaining leftovers after first reheating.
- If leftovers have been frozen, thaw in the refrigerator or while cooking.
- Do not keep leftovers for more than 7 days, if stored in a refrigerator.

SLACKING

According to the FDA Food Code, slacking is "the process of moderating the temperature of a food" in order to properly prepare an item, so that the product retains taste, texture, and safety quality. Slacking is most often used to bring frozen foods to an appropriate temperature before deep fat frying. Additionally, slacking may be used to bring foods that are frozen in blocks to a temperature that more readily facilitates even heating. When slacking foods from frozen to ready-to-cook, it is important that the temperature of the food not exceed 41°F. Allowing foods to slack beyond that point may make them susceptible to spoilage and/or contamination.

DATE MARKING

Date marking is used to indicate the date by which a food should be consumed, used, or disposed. Date marking applies to potentially hazardous foods (PHF/TCS) as well as to leftovers. As with all other foods, these items should be stored at or below a temperature of 41 ºF. If this temperature is exceeded, the item should be immediately disposed of. All foods should be disposed of in seven days (with the day the food was opened being day one) if they have not been consumed. There are certain exceptions to the date marking rule; those include: semi-soft and hard cheeses, uncut portions of processed, cured meats, and commercially acidified dressings.

FOOD SERVICE REGULATORY AGENCIES

Food service is regulated by many agencies. It is important that a facility be in compliance with all applicable regulatory agencies, as noncompliance may result in fines, illness, and even closing of the facility. The following are some of the many agencies that may regulate food service operations:

- Local government
- State government
- Federal government
- Food and Drug Administration (FDA)
- United States Department of Agriculture (USDA)
- Centers for Disease Control and Prevention (CDC)
- National Marine Fisheries Service (NMFS)

FOOD TAMPERING

There are many characteristics of food that make the product attractive to bioterrorists. According to the FDA, some of those characteristics include production of large batches, uniform mixing of items, short shelf life, and easy access to the food. Foodstuffs with these attributes provide a bioterrorist with the opportunity to quickly and efficiently taint a large quantity of food and/or carry out an act that may be difficult to detect and contain because of the short amount of time in which a product is sold and consumed. Moreover, foods with vibrant flavors, colors, or odors are also attractive targets for bioterrorists as they may more easily conceal a contaminant.

Any food security concerns should be reported immediately. It is important that this be emphasized to all employees, and the staff should be encouraged to err on the side of caution. In the event of suspected food tampering, the local law enforcement authority should be immediately contacted for investigation. Next, the FDA Office of Emergency Operations and/or the Food Safety and Inspection Service Office of Food Security and Emergency Preparedness should be contacted on their 24-hour hotline. In the event that it appears livestock has been tampered with, the Animal and Plant Health Inspection Service should also be notified.

CLEAN VS. SANITIZED

Clean means to remove all dirt, debris, and dust from an object. For example, one may wipe a table with a cloth to remove the debris. Likewise, one may clean an object with chemical cleansing agents. Cleaning is a step in the sanitation process. An object that is sanitized, on the other hand, has been made free from microorganisms. Sanitation is achieved through employing either a chemical- or heat-based method. Therefore, items that appear to be clean may still pose a threat of illness if the objects have not been sanitized.

NSF

NSF is the acronym for National Sanitation Foundation. This foundation works to ensure food safety by granting its "seal" for equipment that is durable, cleanable, and can be fully sanitized. When purchasing food service equipment, it is wise to look for the NSF's seal, as it may guide the purchaser to products that will ultimately be safer for the organization and the consumer. Equipment that is easy to disassemble for cleaning and repair purposes is ideal. Moreover, equipment with non-absorbent, non-porous, flat surfaces absent of crevices where food and bacteria may be trapped is preferred to those without those features. The NSF's seal may direct purchasers to these types of products.

CONTAMINATION PREVENTION
PLUMBING FEATURES

It is important that plumbing systems be properly designed and maintained in order to ensure a safe water supply for cooking and human consumption. Certain features of a well-designed plumbing system include:

- *Air-gaps.* These unobstructed spaces in plumbing fixtures serve to prevent backflow. Backflow occurs when non-potable water flows into and/or mixes with potable water.
- *No cross-connections.* Cross-connections occur in poorly designed plumbing systems. These connections may allow contaminated water to flow and/or mix with potable water sources.
- *Appropriate pressure.* When a plumbing system lacks sufficient water pressure, a back-siphonage may occur. Back-siphonages are similar to backflows, however, instead of contaminated water flowing into potable water, the non-potable water is actually sucked into the potable water.

PROTECTING ICE FROM CONTAMINATION

Ice used during food service is easily contaminated by a variety of sources. Some methods to prevent ice contamination include:

- Store ice in a covered bin. Close cover when not in use.
- Service ice with an ice-only designated scoop. Store scoop on the outside of the ice bin (generally on the side) with handle up.
- In the event of a glass breaking in the vicinity of an ice bin, remove all ice and drain the bin. Clean thoroughly to ensure there are no shards of glass contaminating the area.
- Even when using an ice scoop, ensure hands are clean.
- Clean and sanitize the ice bin, ice scoop, and any buckets used to transfer ice to the bin on a regular basis.
- Use care when cleaning in the area of an ice bin. Ensure that chemicals are not sprayed in a manner that may contaminate ice.

CLEANING PRODUCTS

There are four primary types of cleaning supply products. The type is determined by the chemical make-up of the product. Those types are as follows:

- *Alkaline detergents.* These detergents are the most popularly used products and are generally used for structural surfaces and in dishwashing machines.
- *Abrasive cleaners.* These cleansers are used to scour various surfaces and may remove various types of build-up. It is important to use caution with abrasive cleansers as they may scratch surfaces, which increases the risk of surface contamination.
- *Acid products.* These cleaners are most often single- or specific-use products.
- *Solvent cleaners/degreasers.* These products are effective at breaking down and removing grease build-up.

PEST CONTROL
IPM

IPM is the acronym for integrated pest management system. Every food service organization should have an integrated pest management system in place to prevent infestation of various pests, to include (but not limited to) mice, rats, cockroaches, houseflies, ants, birds. Though these pests are small and may seem harmless, they can easily contaminate food with feces, disease, and parasites. Therefore, it is imperative that the presence of these pests be minimized and eliminated, if possible. An effective IPM does not rely on a pest control operator (also known as a pest management professional) to manage the issue of pest control, though all systems may occasionally require the services of a pest control professional.

MINIMIZING PESTS IN A FOOD SERVICE AREA

There are a variety of tactics that may be utilized to minimize pest infestation. Some of those tactics include:

- Maintain clean and sanitary areas.
- Store food off the floor, in airtight, pest-resistant containers.
- Install screens on windows, doors, over vents, and around air ducts.
- Maintain low humidity in food service areas.
- Use dependable vendors who maintain an IPM for their facilities and delivery vehicles.
- Install closing hinges and seals on doors and windows.
- Keep a sealed lid on garbage pails.
- Store food and equipment away from walls.

EFFECTIVE PEST MANAGEMENT METHODS

If possible, the use of chemical agents should be avoided when attempting to manage pests in a food service setting. Chemical agents may easily contaminate food and pose a health risk for consumers. In the event that chemical solvents must be used to eradicate pests, it is important that a pest control operator who is trained and licensed in pest control management be employed. Other methods of pest eradication include using light, mechanical, and glue traps. As with all pest management systems, the most effective means of pest control is preventing access to pests, thereby preventing pest infestation.

SAFETY INSPECTIONS

Safety inspections should be carried out at regular intervals to ensure a safe and comfortable working environment as well as to ensure product quality and safety. A safety inspection checklist may include checks regarding:

- Hot holding and hot food temperatures.
- Cold holding and cold food temperatures.
- Reheating, thawing, and storage temperatures.
- Food preparation surface cleanliness and sanitation.
- Employee safety and anti-contamination practices.
- Review of labels to ensure products are labeled and dated, use of FIFO.
- Chemical checklists, SDS information available.

SDS

SDS (formerly MSDS) is the acronym for Safety Data Sheet. According to standards set forth by the United States Department of Labor, specifically the office of Occupational Safety and Health Administration, chemical manufacturers must produce a safety sheet for every chemical product. That safety sheet, the SDS, must be posted by employers for employee reference. SDS's must be written in English and include the following information:

- Identity (label and list, some trade secrets may be exempt).
- Chemical and common names of the product (if one ingredient).
- If multiple ingredient solvent, chemical and common names of hazardous ingredients.

- Physical hazards of the material.
- Medical symptoms of exposure.
- Manufacturer's name and contact information.

HAZARD COMMUNICATION STANDARD

The Hazard Communication Standard is a regulation enforced by the Occupational Safety and Health Administration (OSHA), an office of the U.S. Department of Labor. This standard requires employers to properly train and inform employees with regards to chemicals that may be used in the workplace. Training should include information about chemical uses and precautions, use of protective equipment, storage of chemicals, how to read an SDS (safety data sheet), and how to read product labels. If carried out properly the Hazard Communication Standard serves the organization as a whole as it may minimize the occurrence of accident, injury, and contamination by chemical means.

DAILY CLEANING SCHEDULE

A daily cleaning schedule is one that lists the equipment and food service areas needing daily cleaning. Each of the tasks is assigned to an employee as his/her area of responsibility for the day. Some items on the list may need to be cleaned once a day, while others may need attention hourly. Utilizing a daily cleaning schedule is one method to ensure upkeep of the equipment and food service areas. By requiring employees to initial the schedule upon completion of cleaning, it also holds employees accountable for their daily duties. It is also advisable that a cleaning inspection checklist be developed in coordination with the daily cleaning schedule to ensure manager supervision over all the areas needing attention.

CLEANING AND SANITIZING STEPS

It is important that all kitchen equipment and utensils be thoroughly cleaned and sanitized to prevent contamination and a possible foodborne illness outbreak. Manual cleaning and sanitization of dinnerware requires a three-sink setup. Using this setup, manual cleaning and sanitization follows these steps:

- Scrape dinnerware to remove loose food.
- Rinse remaining food particles.
- Clean dinnerware in the first sink using warm water and detergent.
- Rinse dinnerware in second sink.
- Sanitize dinnerware in third sink using a chemical sanitizer and/or water above 175ºF. *Note: Using water that is 175ºF may pose a risk of burning to employees.
- Air dry the dinnerware in a clean, protected area.

MECHANICAL DISHWASHING

It is important that all kitchen equipment and utensils be thoroughly cleaned and sanitized to prevent contamination and a possible foodborne illness outbreak. Mechanical dish washing and sanitizing protocol includes the following steps:

- Separate dinnerware that may not be placed in machine and/or requires special attention.
- Scrape the dinnerware free of food particles.
- Rinse dinnerware to remove remaining particles.
- Rack the dinnerware with like items only. Do not overfill the rack.
- Wash the dinnerware by moving rack into machine and following machine directions.

- Sanitize and monitor the process, ensuring that temperature and detergent levels are adequate.
- Air-dry the dishes on the rack.

Sustainability

EXAMPLES OF SOURCES OF INFORMATION ON SUSTAINABILITY

SEAFOOD

According to Seafood Watch, a program offered by the Monterey Bay Aquarium, the most sustainable seafood choices to buy are caught or farmed using methods that do the least possible harm to other wildlife or habitats, and are well managed. Good alternatives are those that may be caught or farmed in less than ideal ways, but can consider buying with some additional information about how they were obtained. Those to avoid are caught or farmed in ways that are harmful to the environment or other marine life forms, or are overfished, which can threaten species extinction. For example, spiny lobster from Mexico is a best choice. Lobster from the United States and the Bahamas is a good alternative. Spiny lobster from Belize, Brazil, Honduras, and Nicaragua should be avoided. Alaskan and New Zealand salmon are best choices. Canadian, California, Oregon, and Washington wild-caught salmon are good alternatives. Farmed Atlantic salmon should be avoided.

TAP WATER QUALITY

The Environmental Working Group (EWG) has compiled a database of tap water quality throughout the United States. For cities with populations above 250,000, EWG rated water utilities according to three criteria: (1) total number of chemicals identified over the past five years, (2) percentage of chemicals detected in city water tested, and (3) the largest average amount of each individual pollutant compared to national averages or legal limits. Among pollutants tested, the three most common are arsenic, nitrate, and disinfection byproducts.

SUSTAINABLE FOODSERVICE PRODUCTS

PLASTICS

The complexity of plastic foodservice products is related to considerations of toxicity in manufacturing and disposal, and plastics variety. The universal recycling symbol (three folded arrows forming the three corners of a triangle) typically indicates something is recyclable; however, the number inside that symbol from 1-7 differentiates plastics' recycling desirability. Generally, plastics with numbers 1, 2, 4, and 5 are recyclable, while those with numbers 3, 6, and 7 are undesirable to recycling companies, and are rarely recycled. The following are the substances indicated by each number:

1. polyethylene terephthalate (PET or PETE)
2. other polyethylenes (PE) including acrylonitrile butadiene styrene (ABS), polycarbonates (PC), polystyrene (PS), polyurethanes (PU), and acrylic
3. polyvinyl chloride (PVC)
4. polypropylene (PP) and ethylene vinyl acetate (EVA)
5. bio-based polymers
6. Styrofoam
7. polycarbonate and other various plastics

Numbers 3, 6, and 7 may create hazardous byproducts during manufacturing and disposal, leach toxic chemicals into food, or contain known carcinogens. These carcinogens include flame-retardants, lead, cadmium, Bisphenol A, phthalates, and other hormone disrupters.

PAPER

Most disposable paper foodservice products are not biodegradable, and none are recyclable. However, several brands manufacture these using recycled content. Two organizations certifying these are EcoLogo and Green Seal. Both require chlorine-free manufacturing. EcoLogo has a greater focus on manufacturing process standards, while Green Seal tends to emphasize using recycled content. While most takeout containers typically contain no recycled content, the Bio-Plus Earth Container from the Fold-Pak company does. Solo, prominent maker of drinking cups, has introduced its *Bare* brand of cups, which are made with recycled content.

SUSTAINABLE KITCHEN EQUIPMENT

The biggest proportion of most restaurants' energy expenses is food preparation, which accounts for around 30% of energy costs. In addition, roughly 15% is attributed to refrigeration costs. These, combined with HVAC systems, water heaters, and exhaust hoods, make up the majority of energy that foodservice facilities use. These high expenses in energy and water costs can be lowered significantly by using commercial kitchen equipment designed to be energy- or water-efficient. Such equipment is often designated by Energy Star labels, or rated highly energy-efficient by the Food Service Technology Center (FSTC), Consortium for Energy Efficiency (CEE), or other reputable research organizations.

Several local utilities and US states have initiated tax credit and rebate programs as incentives for foodservices to buy energy- and water-efficient equipment. Links to rebate programs are available online at www.sustainablefoodservice.com. Refrigeration equipment especially, combined with state rebates, can give foodservices paybacks almost immediately. FSTC has tested, listed, and reported the performance of specific models of cooking equipment for energy efficiency. Steam cookers, holding cabinets, and fryers are among Energy Star cooking equipment. Steam cookers and convection ovens are naturally more energy-efficient.

ENERGY EFFICIENT PRODUCTS

Turbo Pot, made by Eneron, is one example of a line of cooking supplies that saves substantial energy. These pots move more energy to themselves and their contents by having fins that act as heat sinks. The Food Service Technology Center (FSTC) has tested the Turbo Pots, finding they boiled water in half the usual time, shortening total cooking time, and enabling chefs to maintain steady temperatures with lower stovetop flames, saving energy and money. Both FSTC and Energy Star rate refrigerators and ice machines for energy and water efficiency. Although water-cooled ice machines can use half the electricity as air-cooled ones, they use ten times the water, doubling to quadrupling their lifetime costs through water use. A link to an ice machine cost calculator from Texas water expert Bill Hoffman is available at www.sustainablefoodservice.com. Foodservices can install new, high-efficiency walk-in freezers and coolers and plan ahead with refrigeration repair services to procure high-efficiency compressors and motors, since repair companies sometimes stock only inexpensive, standard low-efficiency models.

RESPONSIBLE FOOD STORAGE

In the same way that individual consumer households want to preserve leftovers to eat another time, foodservice operations that prepare large quantities of foods daily must store unused amounts properly if they are to serve them again. This is imperative for minimizing waste, as well as preventing economic loss from purchasing food that will go uneaten. Also, like individual consumers, foodservices are advised by environmental experts to eliminate or at least substantially decrease the amounts of plastic they use for food storage.

Glass is far longer-lasting and environmentally safer than plastic. It is typically oven-safe, freezer-safe, and dishwasher-safe. Dual-purpose glass Mason jars for canning and freezing are designed specially to tolerate boiling and freezing temperatures. They are excellent for storage and attractive. Weck canning jars sealed with rubber rings held with stainless steel clips are becoming popular, offering quick, easy, secure storage. Airtight stainless-steel containers are excellent and come in all sizes. Reusing plastic containers, freezing appetizers or small portions in muffin tins, and using eco-friendly freezer paper or wrap are additional options.

WATER EFFICIENCY

Water conservation by foodservice operations is generally inadequate. Just a few examples among the hundreds of ways foodservices can save water include:

- keeping boiling water covered during slow periods
- maintaining pasta cookers not at rolling boils but simmer levels
- keeping running water, when required, at minimum flow rates
- using efficient faucet aerators and flow control valves on sinks
- cleaning floors with brooms and mops or pressurizing waterbrooms rather than hoses
- melting ice by placing it in dish or mop sinks instead of running water on it
- following best practices for handling grease, oil, and fat
- serving guests water by request instead of automatically
- requesting the local water utility to conduct a water audit

In landscaping, planting water-efficient native plants is paramount. Additional practices include efficient watering techniques and irrigation systems, rainwater collection, and organic gardening methods.

WASTE REDUCTION PRACTICES

In today's landfills, 75% of materials are compostable or recyclable. In foodservice operations, 50-70% of garbage weight is made up of compostable food matter. While the other 30-50% of garbage weight comes from food packaging, these packaging materials make up about 70% of foodservice trash volume. Not producing waste in the first place is the best way to decrease it; this is called source reduction or precycling. Precycling includes selecting bulk food supplies, vendors who reuse packaging, beer kegs instead of bottles, other products that use minimal or no packaging, and products packaged in recyclable containers, such as cardboard or other materials that are more recyclable than plastics. Restaurants can begin reducing waste by conducting a waste audit; www.sustainablefoodservice.com offers a waste audit how-to. They should also train employees in sorting and recycling and post visual graphic recycling guides. They can also implement new programs, such as worm bins, composting, and replacing disposables with reusable, durable, or compostable goods.

In the foodservice industry, disposable products are often undesirable, yet necessary for health or practical reasons. However, more sustainable disposable choices are available today, including products that are biodegradable, reusable, or use recycled content. Foodservices should first reduce the amount of disposable products they use, eliminating any unneeded disposables, and use devices like the Xpressnap paper napkin dispenser to control how many customers take. They can also encourage customers to bring their own coffee cups and adopt reusable takeout containers, such as the Eco-Clamshell.

As an example, some college cafeterias have experienced success with Eco-Clamshells. At the beginning of the year, they charge students a small deposit for this reusable container, which

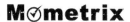

students exchange every time they order to-go meals. Cafeterias not only save money from not having to purchase single-use containers, but also, since they sell so much takeout food, they enjoy very brief payback times.

Management of Food and Nutrition Services

IMPORTANT PROGRAMS AND ACTS

The following acts are important to the food service employee:

The *unemployment compensation program* is administered through the Social Security Administration, and is designed to provide a temporary income to individuals who were terminated from employment. Several factors determine eligibility, and the requirements vary by state. The unemployed individual must have been employed by the organization for a minimum amount of time, and the termination of employment must not be due to the individual's misconduct. The unemployed person must be willing and able to seek employment.

Worker's compensation programs are administered through the U.S. Department of Labor, and are intended to provide disability benefits to employees injured while on the job. Employees are provided reimbursement for any medical services required, as well as compensation for lost wages. Employers are expected to provide.

As it pertains to employment, the *Civil Rights Act* prevents the use of discriminating hiring practices based on race, color, sex, or national origin. Furthermore, employers cannot segregate or classify their employees based on these characteristics. Employers should be careful to exclude thinly veiled discriminatory questions on the application that could be used as a basis for filing a discrimination suit, such as questions about a woman's pregnancy or maiden name.

The Equal Employment Opportunity Act amended the Civil Rights Act, adding more specific language that defines discriminatory hiring practices, and including political affiliation as a characteristic one may not consider in making hiring decisions.

The Fair Labor Standards Act sets guidelines for minimum wage and overtime pay for more than 40 hours worked. The act also sets guidelines for child labor, specifying that children under 14 years of age may not be employed by foodservice operations. Children under 18 may not operate hazardous power-driven food preparation machines.

The Worker Investment Act of 1998 seeks to meet the needs of both employers and employees by setting guidelines for education and training that will help employees succeed in their jobs. Individuals seeking employment will be able to utilize employment centers that measure the aptitude of the applicant and match the skills to available jobs. This also enables employers to easily find qualified applicants for open positions.

The *Family and Medical Leave Act* requires employers to provide eligible employees with up to 12 weeks of unpaid leave to care for a new baby or to recover from a serious health issue or assist an immediate family member with a serious health issue. The act applies to organizations with more than 50 workers, and employees must have 12 months of service and 1250 hours of service with that employer to qualify.

The *Americans with Disabilities Act* requires employers with 15 or more employees to make reasonable accommodations to allow disabled individuals to perform their job duties.

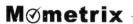

Human Resources

JOB DESIGN

The goal of job design is to organize the tasks contained in one job so that the employee is able to complete the work safely, efficiently, and with a measure of personal satisfaction.

The first step is to conduct a *job analysis*, which consists of an overall study of the nature of the job. The supervisor should seek the input of the employee in this information gathering process.

This information can then be used to create the *job description*. The description is the formal compilation of all duties and skills needed to perform the job. This description can be used to match employees with pertinent skills to a matching job.

The *job breakdown* takes each duty listed in the description, and details exactly how the task is to be performed.

Job enlargement adds variety to assigned tasks to prevent boredom.

Job enrichment builds additional responsibility and independence into a job to add to employee satisfaction.

HIRING FOODSERVICE EMPLOYEES

Successful recruiting can be done from in-house candidates, or can be done outside of the organization. In-house recruiting has the advantages of selecting someone who has shown that he or she fits into the culture of the organization, and retaining skilled employees who might otherwise look for opportunities elsewhere. External recruiting can be done with the aid of advertising, placement services, or college career services.

Employee interviews can be structured or unstructured. Structured interviews are conducted from a predetermined list of questions used for each applicant. Advantages include consistency in information gathering among applicants. Disadvantages include insufficient information gathered from ill-prepared questions. Unstructured interviews use open-ended, unplanned questions and conversations to elicit information. Inexperienced interviewers need to be aware of the possibility of including questions that are not permissible in the interview process, such as those relating to age or marital status.

UNION MEMBERSHIP

A union is a group of employees who use the power of their numbers to negotiate for better benefits, wages, or working conditions in an organization. If the organization is a union shop, the employee must be a member of the union as a condition of employment. In an open shop, the employee can decide whether or not to join the union. Closed shop unions are ones in which the employer can hire only union members, which is an illegal practice. Employers of unionized workers shall not be subject to secondary boycotts, such that the workers refuse to negotiate with the employer via a neutral third party unless union demands are met. Union members may not demand to be paid for services not rendered. Employers may not interfere with the activities of the union by coercing employees or inquiring about union activities. Employers cannot discriminate against union members in hiring, nor can employers refuse to engage in the collective bargaining process.

DISCIPLINARY ACTIONS

Foodservice operations should include a formal disciplinary process in their policy and procedure manual that acts as a guide both for the supervisor and the employees. Well-defined discipline procedures enable the supervisor to respond consistently to infractions, and reduce the possibility of paying unemployment compensation to workers terminated for misconduct. Having a detailed plan of action before meeting with the employee can help the supervisor avoid waffling or backing down in the event of an emotional confrontation.

A common sequence of disciplinary action would include an oral warning, a written warning, suspension, and termination. Each step should be accompanied by thorough documentation and placed in the employee's file. All disciplinary matters should be dealt with in a private setting, and should focus on how the employee can correct or improve his or her behavior. Using positive coaching, exercising patience, and teaching by modeling correct behaviors may salvage difficult employees.

STAFFING

Staffing is the implementation of a plan that is designed to cover all of the human resources needs. In order to properly staff, one must combine resources, including knowledge, skill, and time, to make an organization, its employees, and its processes effective. Staffing includes such tasks as recruiting, interviewing, and selecting employees. Once a potential employee has been selected, staffing includes hiring the individual and providing employee orientation. Then, while on staff, the employee must receive continued training in order to be effective for the organization, and the manager must ensure employee satisfaction, distribution of benefits, and other tactics in order to encourage retention of all employees. In other words, staffing is the total picture, from recruitment to retention of employees.

JOB VERSUS EMPLOYEE

A job is defined as the combination of tasks assigned to an employee, an individual who is hired to work for an organization. The employee is held accountable for completing the tasks; these tasks comprise the employee's job. A job may be performed by more than one employee. Sometimes the employees work concurrently, sometimes the employees are hired and terminated and/or resign one after another. For example, there may be more than one dietary manager on staff at a facility at any given time. Perhaps these individuals split the duties of the job; more likely, however, the individuals perform the job duties during different shifts or on different wards. In this case, there are two or more employees filling the same job. That is to say, both individuals are dietary managers for facility X. On the other hand, a facility may decide that their needs are met by having only one dietary manager on staff. When that individual resigns, another dietary manager is hired. In this case, there is only one individual (one employee) performing the job of dietary manager at the facility.

CROSS-TRAINING

Cross-training is a method employed by many organizations to increase the efficiency and proficiency of a staff. When cross-training is properly utilized and implemented, staff members are trained to perform more than one job. Generally, staff members who perform similar jobs are trained on each other's duties and position. When done well, cross-training enables staff to step up in another's absence. Thus, in the event of an unexpected absence, the facility may continue to operate in a manner that is consistent with prior operating procedure and efficiency. In the event of an employee termination, cross-training empowers the facility to do a thorough search for a new employee as the tasks of the unfilled position are still being completed.

FTE

FTE is the acronym for full time equivalent. A full-time employee works an average of 40 hours per week. Thus, a full time equivalent (FTE) is an employee or combination of employees that make up the equivalent of a full-time employee, or 40 hours per week. So, the number of FTE's does not necessarily match the number of employees. In some cases, there may be a one-to-one match between employees and FTE's. In other instances, the work force of two, three, or even four individuals may equal one FTE. It is important to note that one need not work the standard work week to be considered an FTE. That is to say, any individual or group of individuals working 40 hours per week is considered an FTE. So, one FTE may work eight hours per day, Monday through Friday while another may work ten hours per day, four days of the week. Both are considered FTE's.

CALCULATING FTE'S FOR FULL-TIME AND PART-TIME EMPLOYEES

Depending upon the make-up of the organization's staff, one may calculate FTEs using a variety of different data. See the below examples for sample calculations.

One full time equivalent:

(8 hours/day) x (5 days/week) x (52 weeks/year) = 2080 hours per year

Determine number of FTE's for part-time employees:

In this case, there are two employees, each working 30 hours per week. To calculate the number of FTE's, divide the total number of hours worked by 2080, the FTE equivalent.

(2 employees) x (30 hours/week) x (52 weeks/year) / (2080 hours/year) = 1.5 FTE

Then, to find the total number of FTE's, add the FTE's for full-time and part-time employees. So that, if a facility employs one individual, full-time and two individuals at thirty hours per week, the number of FTE's would be calculated using the information above, such that:

1 FTE + 1.5 FTE's = 2.5 FTE's

CALCULATING THE NUMBER OF FTE'S USING LABOR HOURS FROM VARIOUS PERIODS OF TIME

To determine the number of FTE's for a period of time, take the total number of labor hours for that period and divide that number by the "prorated" FTE. To find the prorated FTE, divide 2080 [the number of hours comprising one full-time equivalent (FTE)] by the portion of the year that is being evaluated.

- For the monthly FTE: (2080 hours/year) / (12 months/year) = 173.33 hours/month
- For the quarterly FTE: (2080 hours/year) / (4 quarters/year) = 520 hours/quarter
- For the biannual (6 months) FTE: (2080 hours/year) / (2 six-months/year) = 1040 hours/six-months

So, if your organization requires 15,000 labor hours every 6 months, the biannual FTE is calculated as follows: (15,000 hours) / (1040 hours/FTE) = 14.4 FTE

If the organization required the same number of labor hours over the course of a year, the number for FTE's would be calculated as follows:

(15,000 hours) / (2080 hours/FTE) = 7.2 FTE

EXEMPT AND NON-EXEMPT EMPLOYEES

There are two types of employees, exempt employees and non-exempt employees. The type of employee determines pay and benefits given to the individuals. Exempt employees are individuals who are on salary and do not receive overtime when working more than a forty-hour week. It is expected that the employee will fulfill the requirements of the job, regardless of the number of hours it takes. On the other hand, non-exempt employees do receive overtime pay when working an abnormally long day and/or workweek. State and federal law dictate the conditions of overtime, to include work hours and compensation for working the extra hours.

SCHEDULING

Scheduling a staff is a difficult but important task. Scheduling must first and foremost meet the needs of a facility. A schedule should be developed such that an adequate work force is available to fulfill the labor needs, without over-scheduling employees. The schedule must be cost-effective and labor-effective. The needs and desires of the employees should be secondary to those of the facility. Obviously, the more a manager can cater to employee preference, the greater the employee satisfaction; however, a manager cannot be perpetually concerned with fulfilling employee wishes. Moreover, schedules should be developed in accordance to facility operating procedure and guidelines. Those guidelines may dictate the length of shifts, number of employees scheduled at any given time or for a specific department, make-up of shift employees (number of managers, exempt employees, and non-exempt employees), etc.

CREATIVELY SCHEDULING

Creative scheduling is a skill that is acquired with practice. Such scheduling is done in a manner that most effectively balances labor needs and minimizes labor costs. Creative scheduling may require the implementation of various timed shifts, staggered shifts, split-shifts, and other similar methods. Vary shift times to meet the needs of the facility. Use part-time employees to fill three, four, and five hour shifts, rather than scheduling an individual for eight hours, which may include downtime. Stagger employees such that start times vary by thirty minutes to an hour. If done appropriately, shift staggering will provide the largest labor force during the highest period of need. Split shifts are when shifts are broken by a period of time-off, so that an employee may work four hours in the morning, followed by a few hours off and another four-hour shift.

MANAGING SCHEDULING CONFLICTS

Scheduling conflicts are inevitable. A manager must always work for the benefit of the facility and that means remaining flexible. Illness, employee resignation and/or termination, unexpected leave and vacation, and other scheduling conflicts will arise. In order to mediate scheduling conflicts, it is helpful to have employees who are available on a per diem basis, temporary and on-call employees are also helpful in filling unexpected voids left by other employees. In addition to unexpected conflicts, there will always be other scheduling conflicts resulting from employee preference. When scheduling employees, try to accommodate time-off requests. In the event that multiple time-off requests are received, grant the leave on a first-come, first-served basis. Do not play favorites; be fair to all employees, and keep the needs of the facility as the priority.

PERSONNEL ORGANIZATION CHART

A personnel organization chart is a chart that illustrates the personnel structure of an organization. The purpose of the chart is to help employees understand the organization's hierarchy and grouping of employees, which enables individuals with the ability to address questions, concerns, and personnel matters to the correct individuals.

COMMUNICATING A SCHEDULE

Most schedules are formulated in a table format, listing the days, shifts, positions to be filled, and the employees filling the positions for the shifts allocated. The schedule should then be posted in an area or on a database accessible to all employees, on the same day and at the same time each week, or how ever frequently the schedule needs to be revised. The schedule must be posted far enough in advance that all scheduled employees will have an opportunity to review their scheduled shifts and so that employees have the opportunity to make personal plans around the scheduled shifts. Without effective communication, a schedule is completely ineffective.

EMPLOYEE ABSENCE AND TARDINESS

Every manager will run into issues with employee absences and tardiness over the course of their tenure as manager. It is important to deal with these instances as prescribed by the facility's operating procedure, and, in this case, guidance in regards to procedure will most often be found in the human resources department. All absences and tardiness should be documented by the manager and entered into the employee's personnel file. Repeat infractions should also be noted. It is advisable to counsel tardy employees in regards to the organization's procedure and consequences of subsequent absences or tardiness. If an employee's absence or tardiness becomes frequent or surpasses the employee's "allowance," termination may be necessary.

MINIMIZING OVERTIME

Overtime is always costly to an employer as laws require that employees who work hours beyond that regularly allowed by law be paid one and a half times their normal hourly wage. Therefore, authorizing overtime on a frequent basis may cost the organization more money than if another FTE (full-time equivalent) were added to the staff. Additionally, employees who work excessive hours and shifts are more likely to experience tiredness and fatigue during the shift, which may result in on-the-job errors and inefficiency. To minimize overtime, ensure that your staff is large enough to accommodate all of the organization's needs and try to have on-call employees available to fill in for absent staff. Use job descriptions, analyses, and routines to accurately estimate the task completion time and to properly schedule staff in order to fulfill facility needs. Also, monitor staff through daily interaction as well as performance appraisals to ensure employee efficiency.

EMPLOYEE INTERVIEW RESTRICTIONS

Employment law forbids many questions from being asked by the interviewer to the interviewee. These restrictions are in the best interest of fairness and to minimize discrimination. Questions that cannot lawfully be asked during an interview include the following:

- Information about a name change and/or maiden name.
- Birthplace of applicant and/or his/her relatives.
- Requirement to produce a birth certificate, naturalization record, or other similar document.
- Applicant's age. *Note: The interviewer may inquire if an interviewee is at least the age necessary for employment. For example, s/he could ask, "Are you at least 16 years of age?"
- Questions regarding the applicant's marital and family status. This includes lines of questioning about a spouse's name, employment status, employer, etc. Additionally, an interviewer may not question an applicant in regards to his/her children or plan to have children.
- Inquiries regarding religion or practices therein.

In the interest of minimizing discrimination, questions about a person's physical stature and characteristics are off limits during an employment interview. Question topics that are illegal to inquire about during an interview include:

- Race or color of skin.
- Height.
- Weight.
- Sex, including questions about gender, one's ability and/or plan to have children and/or use of or feelings about birth control.
- Requirement that a photograph be submitted with the job application/resume or during/after an interview. An applicant may be given the option to submit a photograph.
- Health questions that do not directly pertain to the individual's ability to perform the job duties. Furthermore, women may not be required to undergo any type of gynecological exam.

An interviewer may question an applicant in regards to his/her American citizenship, intentions to become a citizen if not already one, as well as his/her legal right to reside and work in the United States. The interviewer may also ask an applicant whether s/he has the ability to fluently write or speak foreign languages. An interviewer cannot, however, ask an applicant general questions about an applicant's citizenship (including date of citizenship and/or country to which s/he is a citizen), country of origin, or citizenship/country of origin of the applicant's relatives. An employer cannot require that an applicant produce naturalization papers.

Interview questions regarding an individual's education and/or work experience are paramount to determining whether an individual is qualified for the position that s/he is applying to. These questions may include inquiries into an individual's academic, professional, and technical training as well as information about previous work or volunteer experience and foreign travel. The interviewer must be careful, however, not to elicit information that would provide a basis for discrimination. For example, asking a potential employee about his/her affiliation to organizations that may indicate the individual's religious preferences, race, ethnicity, or any other personal and identifying information may result in discrimination. Therefore, it is prudent to avoid asking an individual to list all organizations with which s/he has been affiliated. A more appropriate question would be, "Please tell me about your experience, to include work, volunteer, and other experience that has equipped you to perform this job."

DISCRIMINATION

Discrimination is the act of treating an individual differently because of his/her race, class, beliefs, sex, or any other category. Even if treatment is favorable, it may still be discrimination. Treatment of all individual's must be based upon that individual's merit, experience, and interactions with others. Managers must be particularly vigilant to prevent workplace discrimination, as it is illegal on all levels—educational, organizational, and governmental—and in all states. It is imperative that managers not tolerate discrimination between peers as well as in supervisor and subordinate relationships. The United States Equal Employment Opportunity Commission enforces law regarding discrimination and has stated that ignorance is not an excuse for discrimination. Therefore, anyone with questions regarding the legality of organizational policy and treatment of employees should reference state and federal employee law resources.

BFOQ

Bona fide occupational qualifications (BFOQ) are qualifications, which under different circumstances may be considered discriminatory, that are absolutely necessary to perform the functions of a job. Rarely, if ever, would these qualifications apply, and when using BFOQ as a justification against a claim of discrimination, the qualifications must be absolute. For example, defending that only male physical education teachers will be hired on the basis that men are more athletic than women is illegal. However, requiring that each school employ both a male and a female physical education teacher on the basis that students must have same-sex supervision in the locker room is a BFOQ. In this example, there may be a time when the school is only hiring a male teacher or a female teacher.

PERFORMANCE STANDARDS

Performance standards are benchmarks, which describe the desired work output and outcomes achieved by an employee. These standards should be realistic and quantifiable, such that the employee has a reasonable goal for which s/he can strive on a daily basis. Performance standards are typically developed by defining the standard and the rubric by which the standard is judged. The rubric must be designed such that it provides a clear, objective measurement of each standard. Performance standards should be developed for each task listed within an employee's job description. Once the employee is provided the standard operating procedures and has been trained, it is then reasonable to evaluate the employee's performance based upon the rubric for each performance standard.

STANDARD OPERATING PROCEDURE

Standard operating procedure, also referred to as SOPs, is the facility's prescribed method to address and complete each task, position, and facility procedure. SOPs must be made available to all employees, so that every individual may easily reference the procedure. SOPs are essential to organizations in that they promote uniform policy by which employees may address tasks, questions, concerns, and procedures. Additionally, SOPs are integral to defining and measuring performance standards, which in turn are essential to performance evaluations. SOPs should frequently be revisited so that all procedures may be updated to promote the utmost accuracy and efficiency for the entire organization. When updated, employees should be educated as to the changes to the procedure and new SOPs should be posted accordingly.

MOTIVATION AND PAVLOV

Pavlov's studies into animal and human behavior discovered the effects of "classical conditioning." Classical conditioning occurs when an animal learns to associate a stimulus or behavior with a consequence. Once the association is made, the animal will repeat the behavior and/or anticipate the stimulus in order to reap the rewards and/or avoid negative consequences. Pavlov's theory can be applied to employee motivation, as it is a means by which a manager can reward his/her staff. For example, if employees know that certain actions will be rewarded with praise, time-off, or other incentives, they are more likely to work towards those goals.

EMPLOYEE TERMINATION

Termination of an employee is a delicate matter and should be handled with respect and grace. Generally, termination of an employee should be preceded by documented corrective action. However, there are times when immediate employee termination is warranted, such as when an employee blatantly ignores the rules of the facility, endangers fellow employees or customers, or commits an illegal act. Other circumstances warranting employee termination include chronic absenteeism or tardiness, insubordination, fraudulently documenting time on the job, misuse of the facility's property or resources, an employee's unwillingness to perform functions of the job, and his/her inability to modify behavior addressed by corrective action/progressive discipline. In all cases, documentation of violations to the organization's policy as well as any corrective action and/or counseling that has occurred is essential.

ADAPTING TO CHANGE

A manager can adopt a variety of methods to help employees through organizational change. If employees understand why change is necessary for the growth of their organization, they may be more willing incorporate changes. Some basic tactics that should be employed are:

- Use internal marketing to sell the change to employees; make it an exciting opportunity.
- Consider employee fears and anxieties and address these in the context of change.
- Allow employees the opportunity to share concerns, feelings, suggestions, etc.
- Tell employees what is expected of them during and after the change; describe how the organization will support them (i.e., additional training, accommodations, etc.)
- Ask employees to assist in change process and provide feedback regarding change; likewise, be available to answer questions and address concerns throughout the process.

Finance and Materials

BUDGETING

Good budgeting practices empower foodservice managers with the information they need to analyze the financial status of the operation and make buying decisions.

An *operating budget* itemizes revenue, expenses, debt, and cash flow for the accounting period. This information is used to estimate the profitability of the operation. The operating budget shows the manager how much revenue is required to continue with the operation of the establishment, with wiggle room built in to accommodate unexpected expenses.

The *cash budget* projects the difference between sales and expenses. The cash budget helps the manager predict if additional funds will be available in the event of a crisis. A sound cash budget may also be a requirement of obtaining credit for the purpose of purchasing new equipment.

A *capital budget* is a plan for large acquisitions or facility improvements whose benefits are expected to be realized over a period of years. An example is the planning and financing of a dining room expansion.

COSTS

Indirect costs incurred by foodservice operations are fixed, and remain the same regardless of how much revenue is generated. Examples include the mortgage payment for the facility or fire insurance.

Direct, variable, flexible costs vary according to the sales and production of the operation. Examples include food and paper products.

Semi-variable costs have both fixed and variable components. For example, the electricity necessary to illuminate the establishment is a set cost, but electricity usage rises as cookware is used more frequently to serve larger crowds.

Sunk costs are those purchases that have already been made and cannot be reversed or altered. For example, if a consultant was hired to educate the management team on ways to prevent harassment in the workplace, and the training was complete, this would be a sunk cost.

Differential cost is the difference in cost between two comparable alternatives.

Cost Saving Measures

Food costs make up the largest part of a foodservice operation's budget, but food costs can also be manipulated by savvy managers in order to meet budget requirements. There are many opportunities for food waste to occur between receiving and serving. Using FIFO storage methods to reduce spoilage and teaching cooks the proper way to trim meat reduce waste. Overproduction is common in industries like catering, where large quantities of food are often discarded after an event. Software programs can help managers track waste and determine how much food should be prepared. Combining buying power with other operations allows managers to negotiate lower prices with vendors. Supervising the receiving process prevents "short" orders or substitution of inferior products. Labor costs are not as flexible as food costs, but investing in quality equipment that reduces food preparation time can result in long-term savings. Operating costs such as utilities usually accounts for ~15% of the budget, and are not susceptible to a great deal of control.

Bookkeeping Tools

A *general ledger* contains the history of a foodservice operation's financial dealings throughout the lifecycle of the business. When a new ledger is created for a fledgling business, the assets will include any equipment, property, or inventory on hand, and the liability section will list all loans that were obtained to start the business. As the business progresses, the ledger will be further divided into cash, accounts payable, and accounts receivable sections.

The *profit and loss statement* is derived from information contained in the ledger sheet. This statement lists the income and expenses for each accounting period, and tallies the profit, loss, or break-even status of the organization.

The *balance sheet* contains two sections that, when compared, must be equal to one another. On one side of the sheet is a list of all of the organization's assets, such as inventory, cash, and equipment. The other side of the sheet lists liabilities combined with equity. Liabilities include account payable items; equity represents the amount of money invested in the business.

Analyzing Financial Status

The *daily food cost report* reveals what percent of income was spent on food by dividing daily food cost by daily income. This figure is useful in calculating menu prices for individual items, which usually are priced three times above the cost in order to achieve an acceptable profit margin.

The *profit margin* is calculated by dividing the net profit by the revenue. The *net profit* is the amount of money remaining after all expenses have been deducted, including supplies, labor, taxes, and utilities. A negative profit margin indicates that revenues need to be increased or expenses need to be reduced.

Food cost per meal is calculated by dividing the food cost per month by the number of meals served per month. This figure can be compared to the meal cost for other meals or days to ascertain if the plate cost is reasonable. A high plate cost for one meal should be balanced out by lower priced meals on the menu.

Cost-Benefit Analyses

The cost-benefit analysis is a way to objectively assess whether a nutrition intervention program is desirable by comparing the cost of the effort, as expressed in a dollar amount, to the benefits of the program, expressed in some quantitatively measurable unit. This quantitative analysis can be beneficial in securing grants or approvals to proceed with a planned intervention. The benefits of the program may be analyzed in terms of lives saved, positive dietary changes made, disease status improved, or reduction in the length of hospital stay. The benefits must be expressed as a dollar amount, so that comparison against cost can be made. Therein lies one of the principle drawbacks of cost-benefit analysis; it is not possible to place a dollar amount on a human life. However, it is not possible to execute every program that may save a life, so the benefit may be rephrased as "reducing the risk of death."

EVALUATING PRODUCTIVITY MANAGEMENT

Productivity management analyzes the data that illustrate how inputs, like labor and inventory, are converted into outputs, like meals sold or consultations delivered. If one wishes to increase productivity, one must find ways to either increase outputs or decrease inputs. The ratio considers only one input and one output at a time. To calculate how many meals were produced per labor hour for one eight-hour day, and 12 full time employees were on shift, the number of meals served for that day would be divided by 96 hours (12 x 8).

Work simplification techniques involve examining each step involved in a worker's task, eliminating those unnecessary steps that reduce productivity and contribute to fatigue. The charts and diagrams produced for the purpose of work simplification can also be used in the training of new employees, allowing a new worker to quickly reach the same level of efficiency as a seasoned employee. Examples include process charts and worker flow diagrams.

BREAK EVEN ANALYSIS

Break even analysis is a calculation used to determine the point at which sales volume covers fixed costs and variable costs. The fixed cost of a product includes the total cost required to produce the first product item, and this cost does not vary unless new equipment must be purchased. Fixed costs are high, often in the tens of thousands of dollars. Variable costs are those that are added on after the first item is produced, such as labor and additional inventory that must be purchased to produce each additional product. Variable costs should be below the menu price. Break even analysis can be used to answer the question, "At what point will the production of this product stop costing us money and start making profits?" The answer to this question can help management determine menu prices. The formula for determining break-even point is calculated by dividing fixed costs by the selling price minus the variable cost.

COMPUTER SOFTWARE

Specifically designed, food service/dietary management, computer software is available. The features, cost, and ease of use vary from program to program, so it is important that several programs be researched prior to purchase. Common features found in dietary management software include:

- Meal service features, including ticket/tray-line preparation, payment systems, allergies and drug interactions, etc.
- Menu planning features, including menu-cycle features, creating a visually appealing menu chart, balancing a menu, etc.
- Forecasting features, including automatic forecasting, food-waste analysis.
- Purchasing features, including easy purchase orders, cost tracking, etc.
- Inventory applications, including management processes, monitoring, etc.
- Food production applications, food prep timelines, rotations, scheduling, etc.
- Financial resources, including payroll, cost analyses, etc.
- Safety features, including mandatory reporting information and forms, contamination information, and resources regarding food safety.

REVENUE-GENERATING SERVICES

For revenue-generating services to be effective, others must know about them. This requires internal and external marketing and advertising. Some advertising methods that may be effective include: print media, such as posters, banners, fliers, and signs, in and outside of the organization; promotions, to include taste-tests, open houses, raffles/drawings/contests, discounts; fairs targeting the appropriate audiences; radio and television commercials; web-based advertising. The most effective marketing of any service is done through word-of-mouth, as it is based upon recommendations from previous customers. Offer customers future discounts for referrals. Ask for letters of reference from satisfied customers and add these to the marketing portfolio. Additionally, if revenue will be used towards new programming and/or philanthropic goals, be sure to mention this in advertising. Customers often prefer giving business to a worthy cause versus someone's pockets.

DEPARTMENTAL COST-SAVING PRACTICES

Departments can minimize and control costs in a variety of ways. Some of those ways include the following:

- Carefully schedule employees to ensure adequate but not overly abundant coverage of necessary areas.
- Avoid scheduling employees' overtime.
- Train employees in order to streamline processes, prevent errors and overuse of various products.
- Provide service only during select hours of the day.
- Reduce labor costs by purchasing prepared foods, capital equipment, etc.
- Utilize computer systems to generate reports, orders, and monetary inventories.
- Encourage employees to use products sparingly, if able.
- Offer employee incentives based upon revenues generated.
- Develop and utilize energy-saving procedures.
- Turn off lights and appliances when not in use.
- Maintain insulation around doors and openings of heating and refrigerating units.
- Insulate windows and doors of kitchen.

Marketing Products and Services

MARKETING

A market analysis can help foodservice facility planners determine the best ways to generate sales and profits from their new venture. One of the first steps in a market study is to determine where the facility will be located and what population it will serve. Demographic data in the community can identify target market segments; people with large disposable incomes spend more on dining out. Market strategies match the strengths of the facility to the needs of the target population. Facilities located in areas with high pedestrian traffic or automobile traffic benefit from their location. A competitive analysis can identify competing facilities in the area to determine if the niche is overpopulated. Conservative marketing objectives may include the projected sales for the facility, which factors in projected customer counts and estimated average check. Deciding on the best product mix requires the consideration of trends, customer desires, and efficient use of labor and inventory.

4 P'S OF MARKETING

- Product
- Price
- Promotion
- Place

Product: What is it? What "need" does it address? The functional specs? What are its Features and benefits?

Price: What is Price? (vs. cost?) Channel Pricing? Strategies: markup, perceived value, skimming, going rate. Tactics: Discounts, terms, currency.

Place (i.e., distribution): The Path to the Buyer! Channels, cost (price) tradeoffs, control issues

Promotion: advertising, events, press releases, trade shows, direct vs. indirect, brand awareness, brochures, datasheets, freebies.

PLANNING

The *short-range* or operational planning encompasses the budgeting activities that will take place over the course of a year. The operational plan allocates resources toward the achievement of goals that may bring an organization closer to meeting long-term goals. A sound operational plan can be used as a rationale for the ensuing year's operating budget.

The combination of several years of operational planning can help managers meet their *long-term goals*, usually defined by time periods of five years or more. Long-term goals are defined by their mission and vision statements, which provide the answers to such questions as, "Who are we, where are we now, where do we want to be, and how do we get there?"

Strategic planning also focuses on finding long-range solutions. Strategic planning considers the purpose of the foodservice operation in making decisions that will affect long-term allocation of resources such as expansions, equipment acquisition, or other capital outlay.

NETWORKING

Networking is a powerful and indispensable tool for marketing your business. The more you put into your networking efforts the more you will get out. By exchanging information, ideas, contacts, and business referrals, you increase your client and referral base. You will also find yourself privy to information about industry trends, trade associations, and key people in particular industries.

Trade associations, chambers of commerce, trade fairs, and business conferences offer networking opportunities. Join and become active in those groups that best fit your business goals or match your personal interests.

ARROW DIAGRAMMING METHOD

Network diagramming technique in which activities are represented by arrows. The tail of the arrow represents the start of the activity; the head of the arrow represents the finish of the activity. The length of the arrow does not represent the expected duration of the activity. Activities are connected at points called nodes (usually drawn as circles) to illustrate the sequence in which activities are expected to be performed (also called activity-on-arrow).

WORD-OF-MOUTH

Word-of-mouth is extremely important and is also a very powerful promotional tool. Customers talking about you to friends, family, and acquaintances have much more influence and credibility than any other kind of advertisement.

Remember: bad word-of-mouth travels and multiplies at least four times faster than good word-of-mouth, so make sure your customer service is spot on right from the start. Many small businesses have not only survived (without a huge advertising budget), but grown with good word-of-mouth working for them.

PRICING STRATEGIES
DETERMINING SELLING PRICE

Factor method: The factor method is the traditional way of determining menu pricing strategies, although this method focuses on food costs to the exclusion of labor and other contributing costs. The factor method is determined by first calculating the mark-up factor, which is the figure derived by dividing 100 over the food cost percentage. The mark-up factor multiplied by the raw food cost yields the selling price.

Prime cost method: The prime cost method considers both food costs and labor, and is appropriate for calculating costs for menu items that require a great deal of skill to prepare. The selling price is determined by multiplying the prime cost by the mark-up factor, where prime cost equals raw food cost plus labor cost. Mark-up is calculated by dividing 100 by food cost percentage plus labor cost percentage.

Cost of profit: Cost of profit pricing is used when the menu price must be calculated in a way so that it ensures a specific percentage of profit. It is calculated by dividing total food cost by desired food cost percentage.

Management Principles and Functions

PRINCIPLES OF MANAGEMENT

There is an organization called the Taylor Society that has collected 13 principles of Taylorism, but more briefly, the idea of scientific management boils down to 4 basic principles:

- Scientific research and analysis of work, its elements, standards, and rates.
- Scientific selection, training, and development of first-class workers.
- Intimate, friendly, and hearty cooperation for scientific work principles (anti-unionism).
- Equal division of responsibility among managers in functional areas (not just over people).

F.W. TAYLOR'S CONTRIBUTIONS TO MANAGEMENT

F.W. Taylor is known as the "Father of Scientific Management" and was nicknamed "Speedy" Taylor for his reputation as an efficiency expert. His techniques were:

- To initiate a time study rate system.
- Create functional foremen.
- Establish cost accounting.
- Devise a system of pay for the person and not the position.

MANAGEMENT STYLES

LAISSEZ-FAIRE MANAGEMENT STYLE

Management approach in which team members are not directed by management. Little information flows from the team to the manager, or vice versa. This style is appropriate if the team is highly skilled and knowledgeable and wants no interference by the manager.

OPEN-DOOR POLICY

Management approach that encourages employees to speak freely and regularly to management regarding any aspect of the business or product. Adopted to promote the open flow of communication and to increase the success of business operations or project performance by soliciting the ideas of employees. Tends to minimize personnel problems and employee dissatisfaction.

AUTHORITARIAN MANAGEMENT STYLE

Management approach in which the manager tells team members what is expected of them, provides specific guidance on what should be done, makes his or her role within the team understood, schedules work, and directs team members to follow standard rules and regulations.

AUTOCRATIC MANAGEMENT STYLE

Management approach in which the manager makes all decisions and exercises tight control over the team. This style is characterized by communications from the manager downward to the team and not vice versa.

BLAKE AND MOUTON MANAGERIAL GRID

The managerial grid describes a manager's style based on where he or she falls on a grid with two axes: the vertical axis shows the manager's concern for people, and the horizontal axis shows the manager's concern for production. A manager who ranks high on concern for people but low on concern for production will be viewed as an ineffectual pushover more concerned about acceptance than results. A manager who ranks high on concern for production but low on concern for people tends to exercise an autocratic style of leadership, and is concerned with matters of domination and control. The most effective managers rank high or equally moderate on both concerns. These managers value employee morale and utilize teamwork to accomplish their goals.

TRADITIONAL OR CLASSICAL APPROACH

The classical management school of thought is characterized by the traditional bureaucratic structure of top-down authority. This management style places value in the hierarchy, and depends on rational guidelines to lend structure to the organization. Classical management embraces the scalar principle, which shares that authority flows in a vertical line from the highest to the lowest position in an organization. This school of thought originated early in the twentieth century and is criticized for being too simplistic and not considering the dynamics of small groups.

SYSTEMS APPROACH

The systems approach argues that an organization is composed of interdependent components, so that an event that affects one part of the organization will in turn affect other parts of the organization. The systems approach characterizes an organization as open and interactive, so that the organization can affect and be affected by the environment. The environment could include any entity outside of the foodservice operation that has dealings with the facility, such as vendors or regulatory agencies.

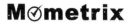

LEADERSHIP STYLE
CONTINGENCY OR SITUATIONAL

Contingency and situational leadership models argue that there is no one right way to manage, and methods that are effective for one situation may be inappropriate in other situations. This theory explains why sometimes formerly successful managers suddenly become inept when faced with a new situation. The manager applies the same techniques that worked in the past, but the results are different because the situation is different. The path-goal theory of leadership provides an example in that a manager may tailor his or her approach to the situation at hand. A strong leader will clarify the path to success for his or her employees, removing barriers and providing rewards along the way. The kind of rewards provided will be tailored to the skill and motivation level of each individual employee.

TRANSACTIONAL AND TRANSFORMATIONAL

Transactional and transformational leadership are two distinct ways of motivating and influencing employees, and each style is grounded in a distinct value set and way of thinking.

Transactional leaders focus on the bottom line, and seek ways to manipulate employees so that short-term goals will be achieved, possibly even at the expense of long-term job satisfaction. Transactional leaders have a limited number of tools with which to problem-solve, but they remain focused on carrying out the prescribed roles the current system has given them, and they are not reform-oriented.

Transformational leaders are concerned with motivating employees by incorporating meaning and purpose into the tasks to be achieved. These types of leaders recognize the importance of building an organizational culture that appreciates the long view. Short-term goals are not accomplished at the expense of employee morale, and managers do not become so mired in daily activities that they lose sight of the mission of the organization.

CONFLICT RESOLUTION

Conflict in the workplace is unavoidable. It can stem from misunderstandings, personality differences, organizational change, or other sources. Conflict can result in lowered employee morale, increased employee turnover, and lowered productivity. Managers cannot eliminate conflict, but they should expect to act as mediators and facilitators in conflict resolution. Managers with a *dominating or suppressing style* may try to resolve conflict by aggressively exercising their power of authority or passively pretending the problem does not exist. Either way results in a winning situation for the manager and a losing situation for the employees. *Compromising managers* try to find a middle ground that the conflicting parties can agree upon. This strategy does little to help the organization or prevent future conflicts. Managers with an *integrative problem-solving style* create a culture of cooperation rather than competition, so that all parties participate in the problem solving. The result is concessions are made without anyone feeling like the loser.

PROBLEM-SOLVING

The nominal group technique advocated by Delbecq is a problem-solving method similar in style to brainstorming, with added structure and control. In this process, a facilitator or leader convenes a group of individuals who silently record their ideas and thoughts regarding the problem at hand for several minutes. The ideas are then gathered by the facilitator, and compiled onto a wipe board or flip chart. Each idea is discussed and clarified for the group. The group members anonymously rank the ideas, and a vote is cast for the most popular idea.

The Delphi technique solicits the opinions of experts on the matter at hand, without the requirement for a face-to-face meeting. Web-based survey tools or email may be used. This methodology utilizes the benefit of complete anonymity, allowing participants to change their minds with impunity. Results are compiled, and an agreement is reached. A second survey may be conducted if no consensus is made.

The fishbone diagram is a way of using brainstorming to determine the cause of a problem in the organization or department, and then identifying and categorizing possible solutions. The spine or leading line of the skeleton is the problem statement phrased as a question. For example, a fishbone analysis may be conducted to address the question, "Why are the meal carts delivered late at every noon meal?" Each possible cause should be drawn as a line attached to the problem statement, and may fall into such categories as equipment, policy, or employees. Possible solutions are then discussed and added to the diagram as additional "bones."

Pareto charts graphically illustrate the causes behind a recurring problem in the department in bar chart form. This is useful when data exists that allow precise analysis of contributing causes. A popular use of the chart is discerning which 20% of causes are contributing to 80% of the problems in the department.

CONFLICT-RESOLUTION METHODS

Conflict in the workplace is unavoidable. It can stem from misunderstandings, personality differences, organizational change, or other sources. Conflict can result in lowered employee morale, increased employee turnover, and lowered productivity. Managers cannot eliminate conflict, but they should expect to act as mediators and facilitators in conflict resolution.

Managers with a dominating or suppressing style may try to resolve conflict by aggressively exercising their power of authority or passively pretending the problem does not exist. Either way results in a winning situation for the manager and a losing situation for the employees.

Compromising managers try to find a middle ground that the conflicting parties can agree upon. This strategy does little to help the organization or prevent future conflicts.

Managers with an integrative problem-solving style create a culture of cooperation rather than competition, so that all parties participate in the problem-solving. The result is that concessions are made without anyone feeling like the loser.

DECISION MATRIX

A matrix used by teams to evaluate possible solutions to problems. Each solution is listed. Criteria are selected and listed on the top row to rate the possible solutions. Each possible solution is rated on a scale from 1 to 5 for each criterion and the rating is recorded in the corresponding grid. The ratings of all the criteria for each possible solution are added to determine each solution's score. The scores are then used to help decide which solution deserves the most attention.

DECISION-MAKING STYLES
THE DIRECTIVE STYLE
- Prefers simple, clear solutions
- Makes decisions rapidly
- Does not consider many alternatives
- Relies on existing rules

THE ANALYTICAL STYLE

- Prefers complex problems
- Carefully analyzes alternatives
- Enjoys solving problems
- Willing to use innovative methods

THE CONCEPTUAL STYLE

- Socially oriented
- Humanistic and artistic approach
- Solves problems creatively
- Enjoys new ideas

THE BEHAVIORAL STYLE

- Concern for their organization
- Interest in helping others
- Open to suggestions
- Relies on meetings

STRATEGIC PLANNING

Practical Guidelines for Effective Strategic Planning:

1. Involve everyone you need to carry out your plan.
2. Work collaboratively with those whose help you need.
3. Schedule a full-day retreat.
4. Document your plan.
5. Make it as simple as possible.
6. Develop an action plan for each strategic objective.
7. Keep the process alive by updating it continuously.
8. Make sure that your plan fits senior management's goals.
9. Don't undertake too much—prioritize your objectives.
10. Keep your plan visual.
11. Communicate the plan down the line.
12. Create an accountability document.

SWOT

SWOT stands for strengths, weaknesses, opportunities, threats. The first two components (Strengths and Weaknesses) generally deal with elements found within the company, and the last two (Opportunities and Threats) examine the environment outside the company. SWOT profiles, along with a corporation's mission and major goals, make up the tools you'll need to develop and form strategies. They are the components of the Strategic Management Model. These game plans reflect in broad terms how, where, and why the company should compete as well as against whom.

ORGANIZATION

Organization Chart:
Graphic display of reporting relationship that provide a general framework of the organization.

Organizational Breakdown Structure (OBS):
Tool used to show the work units or work packages that are assigned to specific organizational units.

Outsourcing:

Outsourcing is paying a second party to perform one or more of your internal processes or functions. Business process outsourcing of certain functions is an increasingly popular way to improve basic services while allowing professionals time to play a more strategic role in their organizations. Frequently outsourced: payroll, 401(k) administration, employee assistance, and retirement planning.

An organizational chart provides a visual reference that shows where employees fit into an organization in terms of rank and functional relationship with one another. A typical chart depicts the owner or department head at the top of the chart, followed by lines of authority leading to the next person in charge, with each succeeding level including the next in line in authority. Chart placement is based on formal titles, and may not be a reliable indicator of where the real power lies in an organization. The chain of command also shows the delineation of authority from the highest- to the lowest-ranked worker. However, placement high in the chain of command does not necessarily entitle one to give orders to one lower in the chain. For example, the director of nursing would not commonly issue orders to a foodservice employee.

The concentric model of organization does away with the hierarchy system, and invites all organizational members to contribute equally to problem solving.

DISASTER PREPAREDNESS

Managers should maintain an updated employee roster that lists names and phone numbers, and employees should be required to wear photo identification badges when working. Only authorized personnel should be allowed in the foodservice department, and visitors should check in with a supervisor before entering the premises. Receiving clerks should become familiar with regular delivery persons and suspicious persons or activities in the receiving area should be reported. Employees should become familiar with emergency procedures during training, and drills should be conducted regularly to maintain awareness. Evacuation routes and emergency phone numbers should be clearly posted. Personal items such as purses and meal containers brought from home should be kept out of the food production area to prevent the malicious introduction of a contaminant. Doors and windows in receiving areas should remain closed and locked unless deliveries are being made. Keep hazardous chemicals in a locked storage area, and maintain strict policies over the possession and use of keys for all secured areas.

ORGANIZATIONAL TOOLS

An organizational chart provides a visual reference that shows where employees fit into an organization in terms of rank and functional relationship with one another. A typical chart depicts the owner or department head at the top of the chart, followed by lines of authority leading to the next person in charge, with each succeeding level including the next in line in authority. Chart placement is based on formal titles, and may not be a reliable indicator of where the real power lies in an organization. The chain of command also shows the delineation of authority from the highest to the lowest ranked worker. However, placement high in the chain of command does not necessarily entitle one to give orders to one lower in the chain. For example, the director of nursing would not commonly issue orders to a foodservice employee. The concentric model of organization does away with the hierarchy system, and invites all organizational members to contribute equally to problem solving.

STAFFING PATTERNS AND FTE'S

Foodservice managers must decide on staffing that will be adequate to cover the production, serving, and cleaning needs of the operation. It may be helpful to rely on industry standards available for the type of operation to determine the staffing needs. For example, in the dietary department of extended care facilities, the expected production norm is five meals per labor hour. School foodservice workers are expected to produce 13-15 meals per labor hour. Managers can calculate the number of meals to be served to determine how many employees should man each shift. Staffing levels can then be adjusted to account for employee skill and meal complexity.

An FTE or full-time equivalent can be used to determine the right mix of full and part-time workers for a facility. The total number of hours worked divided by 40 yields the FTE count. The budget will allow for a given number of FTE's to be hired in a foodservice operation.

Quality Processes and Research

PERFORMANCE STANDARDS EVALUATIONS

Performance evaluations are used by the manager to examine the contribution of each employee to the foodservice operation. The evaluation is a standardized form that allows each employee to be objectively judged against the same criteria. The form can be used as a training tool to let each employee know what the expectations of the position are, and the form can be used as a way to provide regular feedback to the employee about his or her performance in key areas. Employees can also use the evaluation process as an opportunity to give individual and private feedback to their supervisor. Positive or negative evaluations can be used to initiate disciplinary procedures or promotions. Evaluations can be formatted as checklists (yes or no) or scales with assigned point values (on a level of 1 to 5, the employee meets this criterion). Managers need to be aware of the possibility of the halo effect, when an employee's excellent or poor execution of one skill biases the reviewer in the rest of the evaluation.

MANAGEMENT THEORIES

MASLOW'S HIERARCHY OF NEEDS

Maslow's hierarchy of needs compiled research on the factors that motivate human behavior, and then organized this research into a tiered level of progression so that one could understand and predict an individual's efforts to meet internal goals. At the base of the needs pyramid are physiological goals, which satisfy the basic requirements of life such as food, water, and shelter. These needs must be met before one can progress to the next tier, which encompasses safety needs. From a workplace standpoint, this would include the need for a safe working environment. The next tier describes an individual's need to belong, which can be satisfied by the camaraderie found between employees. When these needs are met, an individual strives to meet esteem needs, which managers can offer through recognition of good work. When all lower tier levels are met, one can strive for self-actualization, where one gains the satisfaction of fulfilling his or her potential for growth.

HERZBERG'S THEORY AND MOTIVATION

In the 1950's, Herzberg conducted a study in which he asked employees to recall a time when they felt particularly good or bad about their job. He asked them what made them feel this way, and based on their responses developed his theory of motivation and hygiene. He classified hygiene elements as those present in the work environment, such as pay, supervision, and working conditions. Herzberg argued that hygiene elements could not be used to motivate employees, but could prevent motivation from occurring if the elements were believed to be inferior. In this theory motivating elements are those that relate to a sense of achievement, growth, opportunity, and personal satisfaction. All hygiene elements must be perceived to be satisfactory to the employees before motivation can occur. According to this theory, the recognition and esteem that one gains from a promotion is more motivating than the salary increase.

MCCLELLAND'S ACHIEVEMENT-AFFILIATION THEORY AND EMPLOYEE MOTIVATION

McClelland's theory of motivation argues that employees need a sense of achievement, a feeling of power, and a desire for affiliation. The level of these needs varies among individuals, and an understanding of these varying needs can be used by managers to motivate employees and place them in a position that best utilizes their skills.

Achievement-motivated employees are motivated when they are allowed to strive toward moderately difficult goals. They feel rewarded by the process of problem solving, and enjoy comparing their progress to their peers. Employees with a high need for power enjoy directing the actions of others, and taking charge of activities. A low-ranking employee with a high need for power may be perceived as being "bossy." Employees with a high need for affiliation are motivated by their desire to be liked and accepted by others. They appreciate feedback from their peers and managers about how cooperative they are and how pleasant it is to work with them.

VROOM'S REWARDS AND EMPLOYEE MOTIVATION AS DETAILED IN HIS EXPECTANCY THEORY

Vroom argues that employees will be motivated to perform on the job when they feel that the extra effort they put forth will lead to better performance, and this improved performance will result in the achievement of a desired outcome or reward. The three components of this theory are expectancy, instrumentality, and valence. If the person expects their effort to result in an increased performance, they will be motivated to put forth the extra effort. An employee may not expend additional effort in organizing the stock room if he or she knew it would not be maintained in the following shift. Instrumentality means that the person believes their performance will be rewarded, and valence refers to the value the employee places on the rewards or outcomes. Managers should link better performance to rewards, and determine which rewards employees value the most.

LEADERSHIP STYLES

An *autocratic leader* acts in a solo fashion, making decisions without consulting others. This style of leadership causes the highest levels of dissatisfaction among employees, but it may be effective in some applications, such as a decision that will not be affected by the input of others.

Bureaucratic leaders value organizational norms and the hierarchy present in the chain of command, and expect their employees to respect the manager based on his or her position as a leader.

Participative leadership involves a continuum of participation by the employees or team working with a leader to solve problems. A trend in this style of management is the use of quality circles, which allow small groups of employees that meet regularly to brainstorm.

Managers that practice a *laissez-faire style of leadership* allow workers to make decisions with little or no guidance from management. Employees under this type of leadership tend to suffer from a lack of coherence and motivation in their work.

ORGANIZATIONAL CHANGE THEORY

Several models and theories have been developed that address the need for, methods of, and barriers to ushering in organizational change. It is human nature to resist change, and this includes change in the workplace. Employees may be resistant to change because they are more focused on how the change will affect them than with how it might improve the organization. People appreciate the feelings of security and sameness they derive from their jobs, and may fear that the change will make their tasks unpleasant in some way. The manager should approach organizational change by giving employees ample time to adjust to the change and voice their concerns. Managers may devote one or more employee meetings to discussions about the change. Verbal communication should be accompanied by printed literature, to reduce the chance for misunderstanding. If possible, employees should be included in the decision-making process involving the transition, so that employees feel ownership of the change.

Evaluating Foodservice Operation

Part of a foodservice manager's role is to evaluate the operation on an ongoing basis to determine if the performance of the operation meets the standards set by the management team. The benefits of evaluation include the revelation of the strengths and weaknesses of the operation and the ability to engage in problem solving before issues grow out of control. It is important that the manager document both the evaluative process and the outcome, as the manager is responsible for the quality the department or facility provides. The evaluation may be outcome-evaluated, comparing the end results to the standards developed: Did health status improve? Were savings realized? Alternatively, the evaluation may be process-oriented: Did the process result in the accomplishment of the objectives? Measurement types may include norm-referenced, comparing the learner against the group average; criterion-referenced, comparing the learner against what should have been learned; or comparative, looking for similarities or differences between learners.

Managerial Skills Needed

The management skills required to some degree by all dietetic professionals include technical skills, human skills, and conceptual skills. Technical skills would include those that involve knowing the mechanics of the equipment in the kitchen, or knowing how to prepare all of the menu items in a foodservice operation. These types of skills are highly desirable in a kitchen line manager, who needs to be proficient enough in these areas to both train employees and act as a fill-in worker when necessary. Human skills include the ability to positively interact with others and build trust and motivation through excellent communication skills. These skills are necessary at all levels of management: lower levels of management need them to interact with dozens of people throughout the day, and upper level managers need them to provide a positive trickle-down effect. Conceptual skills include those analytical skills that allow upper management to carry out the mission of the organization.

Successful Managerial Traits

In addition to possessing excellent communication skills, managers should be very action-oriented. A good manager should work alongside his or her employees on a daily basis, and be able to describe his or her day with action verbs: fixing, repairing, regulating, solving, developing, and coaching. Keeping in mind the adage, "The customer's always right," managers should listen and learn from the people they serve every day. Managers should also be internally motivated and autonomous, possessing the skills and confidence to go out on a limb to solve problems. Managers in successful organizations take risks when confronted with unique problems, and explore new avenues to getting the job done. Successful managers recognize the value of their employees, and therefore invest a great deal of time and effort developing, teaching, and supporting their employees. Productivity can only be increased and maintained through the recruiting and retention of motivated, informed staff.

Types of Power

Reward power is based on the ability to reward someone for following orders or the ability to remove negative consequences for following orders.

Coercive power is available to managers who use their ability to punish subordinates who do not carry out orders. Managers who use this power exclusively will never realize the full potential of their staff.

Legitimate power is the influence the manager is able to exert due to the authority of his or her position. Legitimate power is weak as a stand-alone type of power; managers need another type of power to back it up or employees will eventually disregard the power conferred by the manager's position.

Expert power may be wielded by one who demonstrates expertise in an area the other employees do not. Lower level managers with high levels of technical skills, such as kitchen line managers, commonly possess this kind of power.

Referent power is based on personality and respect; employees voluntarily follow a manager with this type of power because they wish to model this person.

QUALITY MANAGEMENT AND IMPROVEMENT

Total quality management, or TQM, is an approach that uses all of an organization's resources to produce high quality products and services. Organizations that practice TQM have the attitude that getting the job done right the first time and every time reduces waste and results in satisfied customers. The three elements that comprise TQM can be remembered as the three C's: customers/clients, culture, and counting. The customer ultimately decides what quality standards the organization should strive for. The workplace culture emphasizes quality in all processes and tasks. Counting means accurate measurement and evaluation tools are utilized to review the efficacy of current practices. The PDCA commitment of managers in TQM means plan what is to be done, do it, check the results, and act on the results. *Continuous improvement* is an important tenet of TQM practices. Continuous improvement is the recognition that one should always be working to improve work processes for better future results.

CRITERIA SET

A criteria set is a series of statements developed by a body of professionals that guide the practitioners in their pursuit of the provision of quality care. Professional organizations such as the American Dietetic Association or the Dietary Managers Association may develop their own statements that describe the structures, processes, and outcomes the organization feels a professional should adhere to in order to provide high quality products or services. The structures discussed in criteria sets may include a description of the quality standards found in the workplace environment, policies, accounting methods, or employee-related factors. The processes described in criteria sets may describe best practices or benchmarking procedures the profession uses to accomplish clinical activities such as delivery of care, or the chronology of events, such as the steps necessary to conducting a successful catering event. Outcomes are described in criteria sets as measurable success or failure resulting from the process, such as improvement in health status.

RESEARCH AND STUDIES
DESCRIPTIVE RESEARCH

Descriptive research involves gathering new data to generate hypotheses regarding causal relationships. Descriptive research is useful when one seeks to study current descriptions of things and explore possible reasons that describe things as they are now. This kind of research cannot establish a causal relationship between variables. The only way to get evidence about cause-and-effect relationships is through some form of experimentation. Descriptive research designs are useful in establishing goals, and as such may examine the question, "Where should we be?" Another emphasis may be on developing methods, which examines the question, "What is best to do?" Qualitative methods may be used in descriptive research, in which observations are described in non-numerical terms. An example includes the case study, which is an intensive inquiry about a single event or population. Surveys are a commonly used quantitative method, which use questionnaires or interviews to reveal descriptive characteristics of a population.

ANALYTICAL RESEARCH

Analytical research allows the study of the effects of variables for the purpose of establishing a cause-and-effect relationship. Clinical trials are a frequently used analytical research method in the field of medicine. Randomization is a basic requirement for any sound experimental design, and this involves assigning subjects at random so that they have an equal likelihood of belonging to the experimental group or the control group. This ensures that sources of variation will be controlled so that no one individual difference, such as gender or intelligence, will influence the conditions of the experiment more than another. The experimental group receives the new program or treatment being studied. The control group may receive the standard treatment, or they may receive a placebo, which is an inactive substance.

COHORT STUDIES, CASE CONTROL STUDIES, AND CROSS-SECTIONAL STUDIES

A *cohort study* is a longitudinal comparison of two populations; one that has a particular condition or receives a certain treatment and the other does not. This allows the examination of situations where randomized controlled studies would be unethical, such as comparing outcomes for pregnant women who received prenatal care to outcomes for those who received no care. Reliability for cohort studies is lower than for experiments, due to the lack of control over confounding variables.

Case control studies examine a population that has developed a disease or condition, and compares them with an unaffected population. This type of research can be conducted rapidly and does not require control groups or special methodology. However, reliability is low because the discovery of a statistical relationship does not infer causality.

Cross-sectional studies measure the prevalence of a disease or condition in a population during one point in time. Such studies may examine etiology, for example the relationship between alcohol consumption and the development of liver disease.

HYPOTHESES

A hypothesis provides the expected answer to the question posed by the researcher's question. A hypothesis is not just an educated guess, it is a rationalized prediction that may be based on the results of previous research, or it may have a theoretical basis that lends credence to an expectation of what will happen. Hypotheses should predict a relationship between the variables in the problem statement. They should not be so far-fetched as to be at odds with all previous research or theories. Like problem statements, hypotheses must be testable. Stating, "Diets in wealthy families differ from diets in poor families" is too vague to be tested. A *null hypothesis* states that there is no relationship between the variables. A directional hypothesis will use the phrases "more than" or "less than." A non-directional hypothesis predicts that there will be a relationship between variables without using quantifying language.

SAMPLING

Sampling allows researchers to draw conclusions about events without having to gather data on every possible event. In the context of sampling, a population is all of the events, and the sample contains the carefully selected events that the researcher will study. The goal of effective sampling is to choose events that will accurately represent the population. The size of the sample depends on the scope of the study and how much sampling error the researcher is willing to accept. Random sampling is conducted so that any one event in the population has an equal chance of being included in the study. Random sampling is not done in a haphazard way; great care must be taken to ensure that all events have an equal chance of being selected. Random sampling is not always possible; for example, a researcher cannot decide to randomly assign some subjects to a group of people who have cystic fibrosis and other subjects to a group that does not have cystic fibrosis.

MEAN, MEDIAN, AND MODE

The arithmetic mean, commonly referred to as the average, consists of a set of scores divided by the number of scores. So, in the number group 10, 11, 12, 12, 13, the mean is 11.6. The mean must be used with caution, because a small number of outlying scores can make the mean less representative of the population. The median is the score that appears in the middle of an ordered list of scores. So, in the previous example, the median is 12. If an even number of scores is present, the median is calculated by taking the average of the two scores in the middle of the list. The mode is the score that occurs with the most frequency in a list. The mode in the example provided is 12. If two modes are present, the data are called bimodal. If many modes are present, mode may not provide the researcher with a meaningful measure.

THE P VALUE

The p value is used to help researchers determine whether or not to reject the null hypothesis. By rejecting the null hypothesis, researchers are saying in effect that "nothing" is not going on. In other words, the data points to a relationship between the variables being studied, and the hypothesis may be tenable. The p value can be thought of as the likelihood of seeing results more significant than what the study achieved if the null hypothesis were true. If the p value is small, or less than .05, research standards state that the findings of the study are statistically significant. The smaller the p value, the higher the researcher's confidence that the results are not due to chance, but are caused by a relationship that exists between the variables.

DTR Practice Test

1. Reasons that the general population is told to "eat your colors" when referring to fruits and vegetables include all of the following except:

    a. The different colors contain different phytochemicals.

    b. Selecting from all 5 colors ensures adequate protein intake.

    c. Doing so ensures adequate fiber intake, which may protect against certain types of cancers.

    d. Eating the colors helps lower Type 2 diabetes mellitus and heart disease risks.

2. Which of the following cooking methods is recommended for cuts of beef such as stew beef, short ribs, chuck steak or beef round?

    a. Pan frying

    b. Broiling

    c. Roasting

    d. Braising

3. Genetically engineering food is a process by which scientists alter the gene make up of certain types of foods to achieve a certain characteristic. All of the following are potential benefits of genetically engineered food, except:

    a. A faster growing food supply, thus greater food production.

    b. Food that tastes better and is more nutritious.

    c. Shorter shelf-life.

    d. Reductions in pesticide use.

4. Egg *yolks* used in lemon meringue pie primarily serve as which of the following agents?

    a. Emulsifying agent

    b. Coloring agent

    c. Thickening agent

    d. Textural agent

5. Which of the following is not an ingredient in baking powder?

    a. Corn starch

    b. Sodium bicarbonate

    c. Cream of tartar

    d. Potassium bicarbonate

6. Two men are the same age and both weigh150 pounds, but one man is 5'7" and the other is 6' tall. What can be determined about their resting metabolic rate?

    a. Their resting metabolic rate is about the same.

    b. The resting metabolic rate is higher for the taller man.

    c. The resting rate is higher for the shorter man.

    d. It is difficult to draw conclusions based on the information available.

7. Which of the following statements is not true about soluble fiber?

a. As soluble fiber is digested, it becomes gel–like.
b. Soluble fiber works to slow the digestive process.
c. Soluble fiber works to add bulk to the stool helps move food through the digestive tract faster.
d. Soluble fiber may help lower cholesterol levels.

8. Chronic alcoholics are most likely to be deficient in the following nutrients, except:

a. Magnesium.
b. Thiamin.
c. Folate.
d. Vitamin C.

9. The end product of sucrose digestion is:

a. Glucose and fructose.
b. Glucose and galactose.
c. Glucose and mannose.
d. 2 glucose molecules.

10. Protein digestion begins in the:

a. Jejunum.
b. Stomach.
c. Small intestine.
d. Brush border.

11. A deficiency of vitamin D results in:

a. Rickets.
b. Night blindness.
c. Scurvy.
d. Beri beri

12. All of the following are true about vitamin C, except:

a. The best food sources of vitamin C are fruits, such as citrus, and vegetables, such as broccoli.
b. Cigarette smokers should consume at least 100 mg per day of vitamin C.
c. Deficiency of vitamin C can result in issues with wound healing, bleeding gums, tooth loss, and leg pain.
d. The RDA is 75 mg for women and 100 mg for men.

13. Which of the following choices indicates nutritional risk?

a. A nursing home patient stable on a tube feeding regimen
b. Diarrhea for 1 week with a 10-pound weight loss
c. A 3-year-old girl with a sore throat and poor appetite for 2 days
d. A 21-year-old male who is drinking protein shakes in an attempt to build muscle

14. A nutrition screen must be completed by which of the following?

a. A registered dietitian (RD)
b. A registered dietetic technician (DTR)
c. A nurse
d. A trained health professional (not necessarily an RD or DTR)

15. Which of the following laboratory data would best indicate nutritional risk?

    a. Fasting blood glucose level of 130 mg/dL
    b. Fasting cholesterol level of 199 mg/dL
    c. Serum albumin level of 3.5 g/dL
    d. Hematocrit level of 42%

16. Which of the following statements are not true about a dietary history?

    a. Information for a dietary history can be obtained using a food diary recorded by the individual for a period of 3-7 days.
    b. A 24-hour recall is the most accurate way to obtain information about an individual's dietary history.
    c. A food frequency questionnaire can be a tool used to obtain information about an individual's dietary history as it determines how often a person eats certain foods.
    d. A nutrient intake analysis is a way to obtain information regarding a person's dietary history when they are hospitalized or living in another situation where observations can be made about the type and amount of food consumed.

17. A body mass index of 28 is considered to be:

    a. Underweight.
    b. Overweight.
    c. Obese.
    d. Normal weight.

18. Which of the following is a false statement about body mass index (BMI)?

    a. BMI is the best way to measure the amount of body fat on an individual.
    b. Men typically have less body fat than women even if the BMI's are the same.
    c. Competitive athletes may have a higher BMI because they may have higher muscle mass.
    d. Although the BMI is calculated the same way, BMI's for children are interpreted differently than that of adults using age and gender specific percentiles.

19. Anthropometric measurements for children should include:

    a. Weight for age, height or length for age and head circumference up to the age of 2.
    b. Weight for age, skin-fold thickness and length or height for age.
    c. Weight for age, height or length for age and head circumference up to the age of 3.
    d. Weight for age, skin-fold thickness, height or length for age and head circumference up to the age of 3.

20. All of the following are true about the Mini Nutritional Assessment (MNA) except:

    a. It is a validated tool used for nutrition screening and assessment in the over age 65 population.
    b. The MNA screens for malnutrition or those who are at risk for malnutrition.
    c. There is a short form to more quickly determine if a person is in good nutritional status and a longer form if a more detailed screen is required.
    d. Specialized training is required in order to be certified to administer this screening tool.

21. All of the following are true about nutrition diagnosis except:

    a. Nutrition diagnosis is when a nutritional issue is identified and labeled.

    b. A physician must make a nutrition diagnosis in order for the individual to receive nutritional care.

    c. A nutrition diagnosis is documented as problem-etiology-signs/symptoms.

    d. Standardized terminology is used to delineate nutrition diagnoses.

22. Potential nutrition diagnoses for an obese male with coronary heart disease may include all of the following except:

    a. Food and nutrition related knowledge deficits.

    b. Physical inactivity.

    c. Excessive fat intake.

    d. Excessive hunger.

23. Potential nutrition diagnoses for a patient with a fasting blood glucose level of 135 mg/dL might include:

    a. Alteration in metabolism (type 1 diabetes mellitus).

    b. Alteration in metabolism (hyperglycemia).

    c. Altered nutrition related laboratory values.

    d. Gestational diabetes.

24. The recommended amount of weight gain for an overweight pregnant woman is:

    a. 15-25 pounds.

    b. 25-35 pounds.

    c. 15 pounds.

    d. 28-40 pounds.

25. Folic acid requirements during pregnancy are increased because folic acid:

    a. Deficiency causes glossitis.

    b. Helps prevent neural tube defects.

    c. Prevents pernicious anemia.

    d. Deficiency causes poor appetite.

26. The best feeding plan for a normal 3-month-old infant is:

    a. (8) 4 oz bottles of 20 cal/oz formula per day.

    b. (6) 5 oz bottles of 20 cal/oz formula per day plus rice cereal added to the bottle at night.

    c. Breastfeeding on demand.

    d. Breastfeeding alternated with 20 cal/oz formula throughout the day.

27. Feeding a preschooler is often challenging due to food jags, pickiness, or the child's attempts to assert independence. Which of the following does not describe an effective strategy for managing a preschooler's nutrition?

    a. The child should be made to sit at the table until the meal or snack is consumed in its entirety.

    b. Small servings of a variety of foods should be offered on a fairly regular schedule.

    c. Snacks and beverages should not be provided within 90 minutes of a planned meal.

    d. The parents should not focus too heavily on what is consumed at each meal or snack because over the course of a day, the calorie intake will be fairly consistent if a variety of foods are offered.

28. Characteristics of the metabolic syndrome include all of the following, except:

a. Serum triglycerides greater than 150 mg/dL.
b. Serum glucose greater than 110 mg/dL.
c. Waist circumference greater than 102 cm in men and 88 cm in women.
d. Blood pressure greater than or equal to 140/90 mm Hg.

29. The best initial nutrition intervention for a person with metabolic syndrome is:

a. Encouraging a 20% weight loss and at least 60 minutes per day of exercise.
b. Implementing the TLC diet and increasing physical activity to a minimum of 30 minutes per day.
c. Encouraging a 5-10% weight loss and implementing the Dean Ornish diet.
d. Smoking cessation and adding medications to reduce lipids.

30. What type of diet is used to treat celiac disease?

a. Gluten free
b. Low fiber
c. Lactose free
d. High fiber

31. What is the recommended initial nutrition intervention for diverticulitis?

a. High fiber diet with adequate fluid and exercise
b. High fat diet with moderate fiber
c. Chemically defined diet
d. Low fiber diet

32. How much protein is recommended for a patient with cirrhosis but without evidence of encephalopathy to maintain positive nitrogen balance?

a. 0.5-0.6 g/kg
b. 0.8-1.0 g/kg
c. 1.2-1.3 g/kg
d. 1.5 g/kg

33. The nutritional priority for a patient with newly diagnosed Type 1 diabetes mellitus is:

a. Weight loss.
b. Determination of a medication regimen then establishment of a meal plan.
c. Establishment of a meal plan then coordination of the medication regimen to match the meal plan and exercise habits.
d. Placement of an insulin pump.

34. All of the following would be potential interventions for a patient with Type 2 diabetes mellitus, except:

a. Weight loss.
b. Increasing physical activity.
c. Reducing calorie intake.
d. Chromium supplementation.

35. A woman with Type 2 diabetes mellitus who is overweight and takes an oral agent but otherwise has good blood glucose control asks you if she can include 1-2 glasses of wine with each night's dinner. The best response is:

 a. A 5 oz glass of wine may be consumed.
 b. Alcohol is not recommended for anyone with diabetes.
 c. It is okay to have a glass or two of wine as long as she omits 2 carbohydrates from her dinner.
 d. She should decide for herself if she wants to drink wine, but if she does, she should take it on an empty stomach.

36. How many g of carbohydrate are in the following breakfast: 4 oz orange juice, 2 slices whole wheat toast with 2 teaspoons of margarine and 1 tablespoon jelly, ½ cup of oatmeal with ½ of a banana, small cup of black coffee.

 a. 50 g
 b. 60 g
 c. 90 g
 d. 120 g

37. Intervention aimed to modify which of the following risk factors will reduce cardiovascular risk?

 a. Age, cigarette smoking, obesity
 b. High fat diet, hypertension, cigarette smoking
 c. Diabetes, homocysteine, alcohol consumption
 d. Family history, LDL cholesterol, physical inactivity

38. Which of the following are examples of omega-3 polyunsaturated fatty acids?

 a. Palmitic acid and lauric acid
 b. Eicosapentaenoic acid and docosahexaenoic acid
 c. Linoleic acid and linolenic acid
 d. Arachidonic acid and oleic acid

39. All of the following are true about trans fatty acids, except:

 a. Trans fats are created through hydrogenation, which is a process that helps to prevent polyunsaturated fats from becoming rancid.
 b. Trans fats are found in commercially prepared baked goods, fried foods, processed foods, and some margarines.
 c. The food industry has begun to alter the manufacturing of many products to omit trans fats, and many restaurants have stopped using partially hydrogenated oils.
 d. Trans fats lower HDL levels and increase total cholesterol but have no effect of LDL cholesterol.

40. A patient in the hospital recovering from a heart attack wants assistance with his menu selection. He is looking to increase fiber in his diet as he has learned that certain types of fiber more efficiently reduce cholesterol levels. Which of the following foods would be the most beneficial?

 a. Oatmeal
 b. Wheat bran
 c. Carrots
 d. Whole wheat bread

41. Which of the following best describes the guidelines for the Therapeutic Lifestyle Changes (TLC) diet?

    a. Limit sodium to 3000 mg/day, calories from fat to less than 35% of total calories, with those from saturated fat less than 10%., cholesterol to less than 300 mg/day, and sufficient calories to achieve or maintain a healthy body weight.

    b. Limit sodium to 3000 mg/day, calories from fat to less than 30% of total calories, with those from saturated fat making up less than 5%, cholesterol to less than 200 mg/day, and sufficient calories to achieve or maintain a healthy body weight.

    c. Limit sodium to 2400 mg/day, calories from fat to 25- 35% of total calories, with those from saturated fat less than 7%, cholesterol to less than 200 mg/day, and sufficient calories to achieve or maintain a healthy body weight.

    d. Limit sodium to 2400 mg/day, calories from fat to less than 30% of total calories, with those from saturated fat less than 10%, cholesterol to less than 200 mg/day, and sufficient calories to achieve or maintain a healthy body weight.

42. Which of the following is the next step for an individual who does not want to begin medication to lower blood cholesterol but has not had success with the TLC diet?

    a. Consume less than 20% of total calories from fat, with less than 10% coming from saturated sources, and less than 200 mg cholesterol per day.

    b. Consume less than 15% of total calories from fat, with less than 8% coming from saturated sources, and less than 100 mg cholesterol per day.

    c. Consume less than 10% of total calories from fat, with less than 5% coming from saturated sources, and less than 50 mg cholesterol per day.

    d. Consume less than 10% of total calories from fat, with less than 3% coming from saturated sources, and less than 5 mg cholesterol per day.

43. The purpose of nutrition screening includes all of the following, except:

    a. Identifying risk factors known to be associated with nutritional issues.

    b. Identifying individuals who are malnourished.

    c. Assessing body mass index.

    d. To more efficiently identify individuals who require a full nutrition assessment.

44. What lifestyle change is most beneficial to a person with hypertension?

    a. Limiting alcohol to 1 oz/day for men or ½ oz/day for women

    b. Lose weight if overweight

    c. Lower sodium intake to less than 2400 mg/day

    d. Increase intake of calcium, magnesium, and potassium

45. As a dietetic technician, you are assisting in a program targeting overweight adolescents at risk for developing hypertension. Which of the following best describes appropriate goals for the program?

    a. Address lifestyle modifications such as weight control, reducing sodium intake, and increasing physical activity that are known to control blood pressure.

    b. Weight loss

    c. Blood pressure monitoring

    d. Teach the adolescents appropriate forms of physical activity in order to promote positive exercise habits.

46. A 45-year-old woman is following the DASH diet. She is consuming 1800 cal/day. Which of the following sets of nutritional goals is appropriate for her based on the DASH diet guidelines?

a. 60 g of total fat with up to 20 g of saturated fat, 70 g of protein, 250 g of carbohydrate, 2300 mg sodium, 200 mg cholesterol, 20 g of fiber

b. 50 g of total fat with up to 20 g of saturated fat, 90 g of protein, 250 g of carbohydrate, 1500 mg sodium, 100 mg cholesterol, 25 g of fiber

c. 90 g of total fat with up to 25 g of saturated fat, 90 g of protein, 270 g of carbohydrate, 2300 mg sodium, 300 mg cholesterol, 30 g of fiber

d. 55 g of total fat with up to 12 g of saturated fat, 80 g of protein, 250 g of carbohydrate, 2300 mg sodium, 150mg cholesterol, 30 g of fiber

47. Which of the following lists best supports a potassium-rich diet?

a. Cucumbers, mushrooms, apples, peanuts

b. Romaine lettuce, pears, walnuts, yogurt

c. Sweet potatoes, spinach, soybeans, apricots

d. Green beans, carrots, pineapple, hard candy

48. As a dietetic technician, you are assisting a 78-year-old man with congestive heart failure with meal selections. He has gained 10 pounds over the past week and is starting Lasix. Which of the following lists reasonable goals for this patient in terms of meal selection?

a. 2000-3000 mg sodium per day, adequate potassium, and mild fluid restriction

b. No added salt diet with 2000 mg potassium and 500 ml fluid restriction

c. 1500 mg sodium, 4000 mg potassium, and 2000 ml of fluid per day

d. 500 mg sodium with 2000 mg potassium, 1000 ml fluid restriction

49. The main, long-term nutritional priorities for post-cardiac transplant patients long-term likely include all of the following, except:

a. Monitoring and managing glucose intolerance.

b. Instituting a high protein diet to prevent catabolism due to steroids.

c. Weight management.

d. Cholesterol management.

50. Outcome measures for nutrition intervention for a patient with chronic obstructive pulmonary disease may include all of the following, except:

a. Improvement in nutritional status.

b. Improvement in activities of daily living (ADL).

c. Improvement in renal function.

d. Improvement in weight status.

51. How much protein does the National Kidney Foundation recommend that a patient with end stage renal disease (ESRD) who has not yet started to receive dialysis treatments consume daily?

a. 0.5 g/kg

b. 0.6 g/kg

c. 1 gram/kg

d. 1.2 g/kg

52. Consider the following 24hour recall for a 53-year-old female, who weighs 60 kg, has been diagnosed with ESRD, and started peritoneal dialysis (PD).

- Breakfast: 4 oz skim milk, 1 ½ cups corn flakes, ½ banana, 2 slices whole wheat toast with 2 tablespoons cream cheese.
- Mid-morning snack: 1 apple
- Lunch: Tuna fish salad sandwich with 3 oz of tuna and lettuce, 1/2 cup canned pears, 12 oz diet cola
- Dinner: 6 oz baked chicken breast, ½ cup rice with butter, ½ cup cooked carrots, ½ cup green beans, 8 oz milk
- Evening snack: 6 graham crackers and a cup of black tea
- Lad data: Albumin 3.6 g/dL, BUN 22 mg/dl, creatinine 1.2 mg/dl

Which of the following statements are true about her protein intake?

a. Her 24-hour diet recall shows she is consuming approximately 1.8 g/kg. It is recommended she decrease protein intake slightly due to good nutritional status to maintain protein intake within recommended guidelines of 1.2-1.5 g/kg.

b. Her 24-hour diet recall shows she is consuming approximately 1.8 g/kg. It is recommended she decrease protein slightly due to good nutritional status to maintain protein intake within recommended guidelines of 0.8-1 g/kg.

c. Her 24-hour diet recall shows she is consuming approximately 1g/kg. Increased protein intake is recommended to achieve protein intake within recommended guidelines of 1.2-1.5 g/kg and prevent malnutrition die to protein losses.

d. Her protein intake is within accepted guidelines for patients receiving peritoneal dialysis.

53. A side effect of chemotherapy is mucositis and xerostomia. This can impact nutritional status because:

a. Weight loss can occur due to nausea and vomiting.

b. Food intake is reduced due to constipation and abdominal pain.

c. Anorexia, reduced food intake and weight loss can occur due to mouth pain and dryness.

d. Weight loss can occur due to dysphagia.

54. Possible nutrition interventions for a child with cancer who is not eating enough include all of the following, except:

a. Serve small meals and snacks throughout the day capitalizing on the times when the child is feeling hungry and wants to eat.

b. Encourage liquids mostly between meals because drinking a lot of fluid with meals may make the child feel too full.

c. Let the child help make the food they will eat and have friends over to eat with the child.

d. Serve meals on a tight schedule because missing a meal will set the child back too far.

55. A 78-year-old man is recovering from a stroke. The speech language pathologist has recommended a NDD Level 2 diet for him. This diet consists of:

a. No restrictions on consistency or texture.

b. Foods that are softer in texture but require more ability to chew.

c. Moist, semisolid foods that require some chewing ability.

d. Puree foods with pudding like consistency and minimal chewing ability is required.

56. You are working at the local health department initiating health promotion programs. Which of the following departments of the Department of Health and Human Services may provide guidance for program development?

    a. Dietary Reference Intake
    b. Healthy People 2030
    c. NHANES
    d. Dietary Guidelines for Americans

57. As a dietetic technician, you are planning menus for a nursing home. Which of the following tools are you likely to use during this process?

    a. Dietary Reference Intake (DRI)
    b. Recommended Dietary Allowances (RDA)
    c. Tolerable Upper Limits (TUL)
    d. Estimated Average Requirements

58. The main highlights of the 2005 Dietary Guidelines for Americans include all of the following, except:

    a. Achieve and maintain a healthy body weight and incorporate at least 60 minutes of moderate physical activity to help with weight management.
    b. Limit fat intake to 20-35% of total calories, with less than 10% of fat intake from saturated sources, and limit the intake of trans fatty acids.
    c. Consume plenty of fruits, vegetables, and whole grains to protective against certain chronic diseases.
    d. Eat less than 2300 mg/day of sodium and consume 3 cups/day of low fat or fat-free dairy products.

59. Which of the following physical conditions would not be a considered a nutritional risk factor?

    a. Obesity
    b. Stage IV decubitus ulcer
    c. Cancer
    d. Fractured femur

60. While serving as a dietetic technician, you are tasked with visiting patients in a long-term care facility during mealtime in order to long-term observe daily food intake. Which of the following observations are you least likely during these meal rounds?

    a. A patient with dementia consumes less than 50% of breakfast and lunch during a 2-day period.
    b. A patient who is S/P major cardiac surgery is not able to effectively use utensils provided to self-feed.
    c. A patient who is ordered supplemental beverages with meals in order to increase caloric intake does not drink the supplements during the 2-day observation.
    d. A patient recovering from a stroke appears to tolerate a puree diet and may be able to tolerate an advance to a soft diet.

61. Documentation developed to facilitate the Nutrition Care Process (NCP) is called:

   a. ADIME.
   b. SOAP.
   c. PES.
   d. DAR.

62. Which of the following is not a true statement about the pancreas?

   a. The pancreas secretes insulin and glucagon.
   b. Pancreatic enzymes are secreted when food reaches the stomach.
   c. The pancreas is one of the organs affected by cystic fibrosis.
   d. Tumors in the pancreas are highly resectable and have a favorable cure rate.

63. All of the following statements are true about the Supplemental Nutrition Assistance Program (SNAP), except:

   a. To qualify, one's gross monthly income must fall at or below 130% of poverty levels or 100% of the poverty level for net monthly income.
   b. Applicants must have no discernable assets or money in bank accounts.
   c. Children automatically qualify for free school breakfast and lunch programs if they are receiving benefits from SNAP.
   d. This program was formerly called the Food Stamp program and includes nutrition education services.

64. Which of the following choices represent acceptable food selections for a mother who is using a WIC EBT for herself and her breastfeeding infant?

   a. Fresh fruits and vegetables, white bread, whole milk, tofu
   b. Yogurt, cheese, peanut butter, orange drink
   c. White potatoes, rice milk, corn flakes, canned tuna
   d. Oatmeal, chocolate milk, eggs, canned kidney beans

65. According to the Stages of Change model, an individual who is trying to lose weight but continues to provide reasons as to why it is difficult for him to make the appropriate changes fall in which of the following stages:

   a. Contemplation
   b. Preparation
   c. Action
   d. Relapse

66. A client you are working with to reduce her cholesterol frequently interrupts you during the session and makes comments, such as, "I am trying to make changes, but I have been under a lot of stress lately," or responds to questions with, "Yes, but..." is displaying what type of behavior?

   a. Ready to change
   b. Unsure about change
   c. Resistance to change
   d. Contemplating change

67. Which of the following is least likely to occur during a counseling session if a client is ready to make dietary changes?

    a. Mutual identification of potential changes that can be made
    b. Preparing an action plan together
    c. Identification of potential barriers
    d. Telling the client what changes need to be made

68. The motivational interviewing style used during nutrition counseling includes all of the following characteristics, except:

    a. Empathy.
    b. Encouragement.
    c. Reflective listening.
    d. Rewards and reinforcement.

69. Which of the following strategies is most likely to have the best nutrition counseling outcomes?

    a. Cognitive restructuring
    b. Self-monitoring
    c. Structured meals
    d. Social support

70. As a DTR, you serve as the evening shift supervisor at a hospital. The food service director asks you to join a collaborative training to learn how the kitchen functions over a period of several months. The training objective is for you to gain familiarity with and competence in the key kitchen positions so that you may better supervise and assist employees. What type of training is this?

    a. Adult
    b. On-the job
    c. Group
    d. Self-directed

71. All of the following are true about diversity training in the workplace, except:

    a. Diversity training deals only with gender and race.
    b. Diversity should be part of an organization's culture so everyone is treated fairly and equally.
    c. Interpersonal skills, on the part of both the organization and individual employees, are an important aspect of diversity training.
    d. Diversity training is necessary even in a non-diverse environment as each individual is different.

72. At the start of a training session, employees are asked to break into small groups and share their 5 favorite musicians or movies. This is an example of:

    a. An icebreaker.
    b. Small talk.
    c. Time killer.
    d. Team enhancement.

73. Which of the following strategies is not recommended for imparting nutrition information to a group of individuals with heart disease?
   a. Provide a limited amount of information at one time to avoid overwhelming the group
   b. Present the information in clear, concise language in the simplest and least complex way possible
   c. Ensure written information is geared to a high school comprehension level
   d. Supplement orally presented information with visual aids

74. The type of menu that provides at least two choices in each menu category is called:
   a. Static.
   b. Nonselective.
   c. Semi-selective.
   d. Selective.

75. Which of the following is not an advantage of a cycle menu?
   a. A cycle menu increases variety.
   b. Cycle menus facilitate staff vacation and leave scheduling.
   c. Cycle menus allow greater ease when forecasting and purchasing food.
   d. Equipment use can be maximized if the cycle menu is planned appropriately.

76. A dinner of broiled fish, steamed rice, cauliflower, bread and butter, and tapioca pudding with whipped cream is planned for a Friday evening at the retirement home. What food characteristic is most lacking?
   a. Texture
   b. Flavor
   c. Color
   d. Consistency

77. The food service director of an extended care facility wishes to review changes in the food served to residents with the DTR. All of the following tools are needed to assist with this task, except:
   a. A diet manual.
   b. A master menu.
   c. Information regarding the number and types of modified diets served.
   d. The production schedule.

78. The concept encouraging a more personalized presentation of menus to hospitalized patients is called:
   a. Printed menu.
   b. Spoken menu.
   c. Menu board.
   d. Master menu.

79. As a DTR in a rehabilitation hospital, you are responsible for determining customer satisfaction with meals. Some of the ways you may accomplish this include all the following, except:

a. Comment cards or surveys.
b. Observational surveys.
c. Eavesdropping.
d. Plate waste studies.

80. Food that is purchased from an instate vendor and shipped intrastate is subject to all of the following regulations except:

a. USDA.
b. FDA.
c. Food and Nutrition Service.
d. All local and state regulations if they are at least the equivalent of the federal regulations.

81. The type of federal regulation that defines bittersweet chocolate must contain at least 35% cocoa butter with a 30-35% fat content is called:

a. Standards of fill.
b. Standards of identity.
c. Standards of quality.
d. Standards of labeling.

82. Which of the following is not essential information to consider during vendor selection?

a. Vender's ability to reliably meet contract specifications
b. Vender's emergency/disaster delivery policy
c. Attractiveness of the vender's website
d. Vender's credit/refund policies delivered products that do not meet specifications (i.e. spoiled or damaged goods)

83. Which of the following grades of beef is the least desirable?

a. Prime
b. Choice
c. Select
d. Standard

84. All of the following are true about USDA grades for processed fruit and vegetable products, except:

a. The grade standards are mandatory.
b. The grade standards are voluntary.
c. Standards are defined in terms of attributes such as color, appearance, character, flavor, odor, etc.
d. Grades may consist of US Grade A, B, C or substandard.

85. During inventory of a community hospital kitchen, a DTR notes that there are 2 cases of canned peaches. He decides to order 1 case of canned peaches. Which of the following is the most likely inventory scenario?

    a. According to the par stock system of inventory, the par level for canned peaches must be 2 cases.

    b. According to the par stock system of inventory, the par level must be 3 cases.

    c. According to the mini-max system of inventory, the safety stock level must be 2 and the maximum inventory level must be 5.

    d. The DTR is basing the decision to purchase another case solely on instinct.

86. Which of the following statements about the receiving process is false?

    a. The receiving area should be close to the delivery docks.

    b. Each delivery should be visually checked against the purchase order and the invoice.

    c. Frozen items should be placed immediately in the freezer before inspection.

    d. Cases or crates should be randomly opened to verify contents.

87. You enter the dry food storage area and make a few observations. Which of the following would be the most concerning to you?

    a. The temperature is 68°.

    b. New orders are being placed on top of existing inventory.

    c. Bags of rice are stored on shelves 8 in above the floor.

    d. An open sack of flour is found in a covered and labeled plastic container.

88. You are completing inventory in the walk-in refrigerator. Which of the following should be discarded?

    a. 2-day old leftover beef stew with a temperature of 40 °

    b. Hard cooked eggs cooked 5 days ago with a temperature of 39 °

    c. Tightly wrapped hard cheese that is 5 months old with a temperature of 40 °

    d. 4-day old ground beef with a temperature of 42 °

89. Which of the following terms means predicting the amount of food needed for a specific event?

    a. Production

    b. Forecasting

    c. Purchasing

    d. Food scheduling

90. Which of the following is not an advantage of standardized recipes?

    a. Customers or patients can be assured that the menu item will not change each time it is served.

    b. Standardized recipes help to facilitate the forecasting, purchasing, and production processes.

    c. The recipes can easily be extended by the chef if additional food is required.

    d. Standardized recipes are necessary when using computerized systems because the reports use that format to communicate to various areas such as centralized ingredient area or purchasing.

91. If you are using the factor method to adjust a recipe that serves 8 to serve 50, which factor would you use to make the necessary adjustments?

    a. 6.25
    b. 6
    c. 7
    d. 0.16

92. Food that is prepared in a hospital kitchen; cooked, portioned, and assembled on the tray line; and then served to patients is an example of what type of food service?

    a. Cook/Freeze
    b. Cook/Chill
    c. Cook/Hot hold
    d. Heat/Serve

93. Which of the following laws apply to a hospital cafeteria renovation?

    a. The Rehabilitation Act
    b. The Workforce Investment Act
    c. The Civil Service Reform Act
    d. The Americans with Disabilities Act

94. An individual has become ill 6 hours after eating at a salad bar buffet containing various cooked meats, cottage cheese, and potato salad. The symptoms are nausea, vomiting, diarrhea, and severe abdominal cramping. The microorganism most likely responsible for this outbreak is:

    a. Clostridium botulinum.
    b. Staphylococcus aureus.
    c. E. coli 0157:H7.
    d. Campylobacter jejuni.

95. As the cafeteria manager, you notice that the hamburgers are not cooked to the proper temperature and are very rare on the inside. What are you most concerned about?

    a. Salmonella
    b. E. coli 0157:H7
    c. Bacillus cereus
    d. Shigella

96. Which of the following groups are at the highest risk if listeriosis is contracted?

    a. Infants
    b. Children, aged 1-5
    c. Older adults
    d. Pregnant women

97. Which of the following temperature ranges is known as the danger zone?

    a. 41-140 °F
    b. 35-145°F
    c. 50-150°F
    d. 40-120°F

98. A famous television star is admitted to a hospital due to an injury that occurred during filming. Many employees have legitimate access to his computerized medical record, but some who do not, access his records anyways. Later, information is leaked to tabloids. A review of who has authorized access occurs, and many employees are terminated. What is a possible reason for termination?

    a.   Violation of doctor- patient confidentiality
    b.   Violation of freedom of speech
    c.   Violation of HIPAA
    d.   Violation of FERPA

99. As the evening supervisor in the kitchen of a small nursing home, it is your job to verify the dish machine is operating correctly. Which of the following would concern you?

    a.   Wash temperature of 140°F
    b.   Rinse temperature of 165°F
    c.   Dishes drying on racks to allow for air drying
    d.   Prewash water temperature of 120°F

100. A food service aide has complained to you about frequently finding bloody tissues on one patient's meal tray. How do you correct this?

    a.   Tell the employee to remove the tissue and place them in trash can.
    b.   The employee should refuse to remove the tray from the room.
    c.   Tell the employee not to worry and remove the tray from the room.
    d.   Speak to the nurse about the situation so the tissue can be properly disposed. The employee should wear gloves to remove the tray form the room.

101. Which of the following types of fire extinguishers should not be used on a grease fire?

    a.   Foam
    b.   Sodium bicarbonate
    c.   Water
    d.   Carbon dioxide

102. A woman and a man both interview for a cashier position in a hospital cafeteria. Both are hired for the job but the woman is paid $1.00 less per hour than the man. Identify the law that may be violated.

    a.   Fair Labor Standards Act
    b.   Equal Pay Act
    c.   Minimum Wage Act
    d.   Fair Pay Act

103. Which of the following individuals is likely eligible for unemployment compensation under the Social Security Act of 1935?

    a.   A tray-line worker who has been dismissed due to workforce reduction
    b.   A cook who was using recreational drugs in the restroom during scheduled breaks
    c.   A DTR who voluntarily stopped showing up for work.
    d.   A food service supervisor who has accepted a job requiring early morning hours but habitually comes in 1 hour late each day

104. Which of the following employment advertisement modes is least likely to effectively recruit a new food service director at a large, tertiary-care hospital?

    a. Internet advertising on a Web site, such as Monster.com or careerbuilder.com

    b. Internal sources

    c. Recruitment agency

    d. Advertising in a weekly local newspaper

105. Retaining good employees is challenging. Which of the following is least likely to promote employee retention?

    a. Offering an excellent benefits package, including health insurance, life insurance, 401K, etc.

    b. Rewarding employees for good performance with bonuses or consistent raises

    c. Maintaining rigid scheduling because work comes first

    d. Providing opportunities to learn new skills

106. A new dish machine is needed for the retirement home kitchen. The money to purchase this piece of equipment will come from which part of the budget?

    a. Master

    b. Operating

    c. Capital

    d. Cash

107. Labor costs in the hospital cafeteria have been over budget for several months due to overtime. Which of the following would not be an immediate solution to the problem?

    a. Dismiss a few employees to control labor costs

    b. Review the operation to see if additional self-serve stations can be implemented

    c. Review the scheduling procedure to see if overtime is justified and see if some of the prep work can be moved to non-peak hours

    d. Determine if employees are being properly supervised and performing tasks appropriately

108. In Maslow's Hierarchy of needs, which of the following needs must be met first?

    a. Social

    b. Safety

    c. Self-esteem

    d. Physiological

109. An employee attempts to provide input to his food service manager with regard to the workflow surrounding the prep area. The manager tells the employee that the necessary changes have already been instituted and there is no room for discussion on the matter. This is an example of what type of leadership style?

    a. Democratic

    b. Autocratic

    c. Bureaucratic

    d. Participative

110. Effective communication involves all of the following, except:

    a. Oral

    b. Written

    c. Action or demonstration

    d. Grapevine

111. Which of the following would not be an example of good merchandising?

a. Fruit in a plastic container in the refrigerator
b. Polished, clean, and unbruised apples, oranges, pears, and bananas in a large wicker basket
c. Pre-plated fruit plates with interesting garnishes
d. Weekly-featured fresh fruits with recipes, creative presentation of the fruit, such as ka-bobs, or a special fruit dip

112. The hospital cafeteria has added Pizza Hut pizza and Boar's Head deli meats to its employee menu. This is an example of:

a. Marketing
b. Branding
c. Promotion planning
d. Mark-up merchandising

113. Which of the following is not a JCAHO approved medical abbreviation?

a. mg for milligram
b. ml for milliliter
c. Q.D. for every day or daily
d. IV for intravenous

114. As a newly hired DTR in charge of the cafeteria, you are asked to participate in a food safety program sponsored by the National Restaurant Association. The name of this program is:

a. Federal Food Safety Program
b. Food Safety Certificate Program
c. iPura Food Safety
d. ServSafe

115. Which of the following scenarios would not raise red flags to a food service manager?

a. A food service worker has a broken washing machine and has not had time to go to the laundromat to clean his uniforms.
b. A food service worker comes to work without a fever but complains of allergies and congestion.
c. A food service employee making sandwiches in the deli is sneezing frequently and often forgets to sneeze into her elbow.
d. A cafeteria line server absentmindedly touches her head and face when no customers are being served.

116. A health inspector visits the hospital food service operation where you are a food service supervisor. As the only supervisor on duty at the time, which of the following should you not do during the inspection?

a. Ask to see the inspector's credentials
b. Follow the inspector throughout the inspection, make notes of any violations found, and try to fix any small problems while the inspector is there
c. Sign the copy of the inspection
d. Refuse the inspection on the grounds that a manager level employee is not present for the inspection

117. Which of the following is not addressed in the FDA Food Code?
- a. Food service establishment flooring material characteristics
- b. Specific dress code policies for food service personnel working in kitchens
- c. Guideline for using ice to keep foods cool
- d. Guideline for sinks used for hand washing

118. The Joint Commission on the Accreditation of Healthcare Organizations (JCAHO) uses which of the following to assess patient care during a survey?
- a. Tracer Methodology
- b. Chart review
- c. Audits
- d. Standards interpretation

119. The Joint Commission on the Accreditation of Healthcare Organizations (JCAHO) has implemented patient safety goals. All of the following are part of these goals, except:
- a. The use of 2 patient identifiers.
- b. Prevention of decubitus ulcers.
- c. Improvement in the safety of all medications.
- d. Improvement in the communication between healthcare providers.

120. Which of the following is the term that means comparing one's performance with the performance of another?
- a. Outcomes management
- b. Benchmarking
- c. Performance outcome
- d. Resource measurement

121. In the quality improvement process, which of the following is a difficult outcome to measure?
- a. The percentage of patients who had a nutrition screening completed within 24 hours of admission
- b. The number of patients who had a nutrition consult triggered because of low serum albumin on admission
- c. The percentage of patients who met 75% of their nutrient goals everyday
- d. The percentage of patients receiving nutrition support through the most appropriate route

122. The Institute of Medicine has identified 6 Quality Aims. These include all of the following, except:
- a. Patient Safety and Timeliness.
- b. Patient-Centered and Equity.
- c. Effectiveness and Efficiency.
- d. Competency and Relevance.

123. Which of the following is not a true statement about the American Dietetic Association's Standards of Professional Performance?

a. The standards apply only to RDs.
b. The standards apply to all RDs and DTRs.
c. The standards were written based on specific training levels of RDs and DTRs as well as the level of responsibility of each.
d. The standards address 6 areas of professional behavior, including communication and quality of practice.

124. The DTR at the local community hospital is busy with nutrition screening, assessment, documentation, and education. The RD position has been vacant for quite a few months with no immediate prospects. The Director of Nutrition and Food Services feels the DTR is doing a great job. Is there a need to be concerned?

a. No, the important point is that the patients are receiving nutritional care.
b. Yes, the DTR should be completing just the nutrition screens.
c. No, the state regulations do not specify the work must be done by an RD.
d. Yes, the DTR is working without an RD's supervision and is putting the hospital at risk for consequences, such as fines or loss of license.

125. All of the following maybe tasks performed by a DTR under the supervision of a RD, except:

a. Completing nutrition screens in the retirement home.
b. Teaching nutrition education classes at WIC.
c. Providing tube feeding recommendations on the RD's day off.
d. Working at a fitness club assisting with weight loss.

126. The American Dietetic Association and the Commission on Dietetic Registration (CDR) have written a Code of Ethics. Which of the following is an example of an ethics violation?

a. The hospital food service receives holiday cards from food vendors.
b. The inpatient RD accepts monetary gifts from a holistic physicians' group and in return, is advising patients to purchase the products offered by this group.
c. The DTR is taking diet histories on all new admissions.
d. The DTR in a long-term care setting was recently in a car accident. While on a medical leave of absence, he became addicted to pain killers but has since received treatment for this addiction and is in recovery.

127. A patient you are working with reads various magazines, many of which focus on health and nutrition. She has many questions regarding what she is reading as the advice seems conflicting. All of the following would be appropriate responses, except:

a. Asking her to determine whether the article is reporting information and advocating change based on information from only one study.
b. Asking her if you may look at the article in order to determine how the diet was evaluated.
c. Telling her that if it is published in most magazines, the information must be correct.
d. Asking her if the article was reporting on a study done on animals or people. Also, ask her how large the sample size was.

128. You are asked to give a presentation at the senior center on new advances in nutrition and heart disease. When reviewing the literature, the best type of studies to review is:

a. Randomized control trials.
b. Cohort studies.
c. Case controlled studies.
d. Consensus statements.

129. As a DTR, part of your job is to complete the initial nutrition screening on all admissions. Next, you collaborate with the RD to decide how the department tasks will be completed. You have a good working relationship with the RD. The Clinical Nutrition Manager asks the RD for input on your performance over the past year. A reason for this may be:

a. She is getting ready to perform corrective discipline.
b. She is getting ready to complete your performance appraisal.
c. She is trying to keep tabs on the inpatient staff.
d. She is trying to write a job description.

Answer Key and Explanations

1. B: "Eat your Colors" is a mnemonic phrase used to remind the general population to select a variety of fruits and vegetables based on colors. The color groups are red, yellow/orange, green, purple/blue, and tan/white. Eating a variety of colors ensures consumption of a wide range of vitamins and minerals. Fruits and vegetables are excellent sources of phytochemicals, which fight disease. Increasing fruit and vegetable consumption may reduce the risk of cancer, Type 2 diabetes mellitus, and heart disease. Fruits and vegetables are naturally low in fat but may not necessarily supply enough protein in the diet. They are excellent sources of fiber as well.

2. D: Cuts of meat, such as stew beef, short ribs, chuck steak, beef round, or pot roast are usually less tender cuts and require a moist method of cooking to improve tenderness. Braising typically requires that the meat be browned in a hot frying pan with a little bit of oil to seal in the juices. Liquid, such as water or broth, is then added to the pan. The lid is placed on tightly, and the meat is cooked slowly over a period of time until the meat is tender and done. Roasting, broiling, and pan-frying work better for cuts of meat that are already tender and flavorful.

3. C: Genetically engineered food is a fast-growing industry. Scientists alter the genetic makeup of foods to induce a certain trait without having to wait for natural evolution. Scientists support genetic engineering saying that the potential benefits include more nutritious and flavorful food as well as faster growing periods, which results in faster food production. Increases in food shelf-life may also be a result of genetic engineering. Pesticide use is reduced; however, genetic engineering may affect the resistance of plants to certain pests. Foods that have been genetically engineered include potatoes, tomatoes, and soybeans. Animals are also subject to this process. There are still a number of unknowns about genetic engineering, such as the effects of genetically engineered foods on children and the potential risks for allergic reactions, which make people question whether this process is safe for the long-term.

4. B: Typically egg yolks serve as a coloring agent in lemon meringue pie (lemon does not provide the same rich yellow color). As a whole, eggs also act as emulsifying agents (the lecithin forms a protective layer around lipid particles); thickening agents (the egg yolks act as a binding agent when heated); and textural agents. As the protein in eggs is denatured, it becomes rigid, yet it also has a rubbery, elastic quality to it as well. Egg whites can be beaten until foamy, which will then add texture to products such as soufflés, omelets, and angel food cake.

5. D: Baking powder is a leavening agent for baked products. Baking powder consists of 3 ingredients: baking soda, cream of tartar, and corn starch. The baking soda acts as the alkaline salt, the cream of tartar acts as the acidic salt, and the corn starch absorbs moisture. Ultimately, baking powder produces carbon dioxide. Baking powder available in two forms: single and double acting. Single acting baking powder is activated by moisture in the recipe. Recipes using this form need to be baked immediately because the reaction starts right away. Double acting baking powder works in two phases. The first reaction occurs while at room temperature, and the second occurs in the oven. Generally baking powder is used in cake and biscuit recipes while baking soda is used in cookies.

6. B: The resting metabolic rate (RMR) is the amount of calories required to maintain bodily functions, such as breathing and maintenance of temperature. The RMR is usually 10-20% higher than the basal metabolic rate, which allows for the thermic effect of food (TEF). RMR is affected by many factors such as age, sex, body size, and composition. Typically, if two men weigh the same but

146

have different heights, the taller man will have a higher RMR because his surface area is greater. In terms of body composition, a higher percentage of lean body mass will produce a higher metabolic rate. Women tend to have lower metabolic rates than men. As one ages, the metabolic rate decreases. Hormonal status and fever also affect the RMR.

7. C: There are two types of fiber found in foods: soluble and insoluble. Soluble fiber is found in foods such as oat bran, legumes, fruits, and vegetables. The addition of soluble fiber to one's diet has been shown to help lower cholesterol levels. Once it is consumed and comes in contact with water, it forms a gel-like substance. Soluble fiber works to slow the digestive process. Insoluble fiber, on the other hand, works to slow the transit of food through the digestive tract because it adds bulk to the stool. Adding insoluble fiber is helpful when treating constipation. Whole grain breads and cereals as well as fruits and vegetables contain insoluble fiber.

8. D: Individuals with chronic alcohol abuse are at risk for many vitamin or mineral deficiencies even if they are well nourished. Chronic alcohol abusers may experience a folate deficiency, which may lead to anemia, because alcohol interferes with the metabolism of folate. Thiamin is another potential deficiency directly related to alcohol abuse. This leads to Wernicke-Korsakoff Syndrome, which is characterized by confusion, memory loss, and problems with coordination. It can lead to permanent brain damage. Other B vitamins may also be affected by alcohol abuse. Magnesium is another nutrient that is commonly deficient in those with excessive alcohol intake. Other nutrients may also be affected depending upon the individual's diet and overall nutritional status.

9. A: Sucrose is an example of a disaccharide. Sucrose is commonly referred to as table sugar and is found in other food products, such as maple syrup and molasses. When sucrose is consumed, it is hydrolyzed by sucrase into glucose and fructose when a water molecule splits in the digestive process. Both glucose and fructose are monosaccharides. Other disaccharides include maltose, which is broken down by maltase into 2 glucose molecules, and lactose, which is broken down by lactase into glucose and galactose. Glucose is then used for energy by the brain and also provides energy for muscles and tissue. Glucose can be stored for the short-term as glycogen. Insulin and glucagon work to maintain a normal blood glucose level in the absence of diabetes.

10. B: Protein digestion initially starts in the stomach; however, the duodenum is the major site of protein digestion. Enzymes such as pancreatic trypsin or chymotrypsin work to break intact protein down into smaller polypeptides and amino acids. Enzymes, such as proteolytic peptidases, located on the brush border also help digest protein. Small peptides can be absorbed as is but dipeptides need to be further reduced to amino acids. It is here on the brush border that the final phase of protein digestion occurs. The majority of protein absorption occurs before it gets to the jejunum so minimal protein is wasted and excreted.

11. A: The incidence of vitamin D deficiency is increasing. It may present as rickets in children or osteomalacia in adults. Rickets occurs because bone mineralization is damaged. Rickets can also result from a calcium or phosphorus deficiency. Vitamin D deficiency can occur because there is not sufficient exposure to sunlight or from a lack of dietary sources. Vitamin D deficiency can also occur due to issues with lipid malabsorption or kidney disorders. Individuals who are at the highest risk for developing vitamin D deficiencies include the elderly and infants who are exclusively breastfed. A deficiency can be determined by having a level of 25-hydroxy-vitamin D less than 50 mg/ml. The best food sources of vitamin D include fortified dairy products, fish, eggs, and cod liver oil.

12. D: The RDA for vitamin C is 75 mg for women over the age of 19, however, the amount increases if the woman is pregnant or breastfeeding. Pregnancy increases vitamin C requirements to 85 mg/day for ages over 19, and lactating women over age 19 require 120 mg/day. The RDA for men is 90 mg/day. Smokers do need additional vitamin C over and above the RDA because they typically have lower serum levels of the nutrient. Deficiency of vitamin C is called scurvy, and this may be characterized by swollen and bleeding gums, tooth loss as well as fatigue, skin lesions, and leg pain. Vitamin C deficiency can also negatively impact wound healing. The best sources of vitamin C are citrus fruits, strawberries, and cantaloupe; and vegetables, such as broccoli, peppers, and Brussels sprouts.

13. B: A person experiencing diarrhea for a period of 1 week and who has had a 10-pound weight loss is at a nutritional risk requires immediate attention. A patient who is stable on tube feeding is not at nutritional risk, however, if the patient was losing weight, had poor skin integrity, or was not receiving the full tube feeding prescription regularly, that individual would then be at risk. A 3-year-old with a poor appetite and a sore throat is not necessarily a nutritional risk unless the difficulty with swallowing persisted and was unrelated to a minor viral or bacterial illness. A 21-year-old who is drinking protein shakes to build muscle would not be considered at nutritional risk unless the amount of protein he is taking in is adversely affecting kidney or liver function or has other risk factors.

14. D: A nutrition screen can be completed by either a registered dietitian (RD) or a registered dietetic technician (DTR), but in many places, the screening is done by a trained health professional such as a nurse or physician. Nutrition screening is done in a hospital setting; however, it is also done in settings such as clinics, senior centers, or in the individual's home. If the individual is identified as high risk, he or she is then referred to an RD. In many institutions, it is within the DTR's scope of practice to do the nutrition screening.

15. A: There are many different laboratory tests that can be used for nutritional screening purposes. Fasting blood glucose (FBG) level is a useful test as it can identify diabetes or other blood glucose issues. A normal FBG is 70-99 mg/dL. A level between 100-125 mg/dL may indicate prediabetes and over 126 mg/dL indicates diabetes. A level of 126 mg/dL is a significant nutritional risk factor. Fasting serum cholesterol is not technically high at 199 mg/dL but should be evaluated along with other lipid tests such as HDL, LDL, and triglycerides. A serum albumin of 3.5 g/dL is considered normal. A lower level may indicate visceral protein depletion. A hematocrit of 42% is also normal and a lower level may be indicative of anemia and is a nutritional risk factor. Other laboratory values that may be used for nutrition screening include renal labs, such as BUN, and creatinine or electrolyte tests.

16. B: A dietary history involves obtaining information about the type of food a person eats, food patterns, and quantities of food. There are many ways to obtain this information. A 24-hour recall is helpful, but it may not always be the most accurate as the person may not eat his/her typical diet and/or may struggle to accurately recall all food consumed. A food diary is often used to record what a person eats and generally can be kept for a period of 3-7 days. It may incorporate a weekend day as well. A food frequency questionnaire can also be used to help determine a person's eating habits, such as the most frequently consumed food and beverage groups. A nutrient intake analysis is also referred to as a calorie count and is often used in a hospital setting but may not always be accurate.

17. B: Body mass index (BMI) is a validated tool to help determine nutritional status. A BMI requires a height and a weight value, which when inputted in a formula, can determine a person's weight status. The metric formula is: BMI = weight (kg) ÷ height (m)^2. It is an inexpensive tool that is easily used by clinicians as well as the average person. BMI is classification is as follows: underweight if less than 18.5 kg/m^2, overweight between 25-29.9 kg/m^2, and obese greater than 30 kg/m². BMI values tend to rise as a person ages due to changes in overall body composition as well as changes in weight. Normal weight is considered to be 18.5-24.9.

18. A: Body mass index (BMI) is not the best way to determine a person's body mass. BMI takes into account both fat and muscle mass and is not able to differentiate between these. Women typically have higher amounts of fat than men do even if the BMI is the same. Older adults also typically have more body fat than younger people. Competitive athletes may have a higher BMI because of increased muscle mass. This needs to be taken into account when interpreting the BMI value. BMI is calculated the same way for children; however, the BMI should not be interpreted using adult data. Gender and age specific percentiles have been established and should be utilized.

19. C: Anthropometric measurements in children are extremely important as a way to monitor adequacy of growth. For infants up to the age of 3, weight for age, length for age and head circumference should be measured and recorded on a growth chart. Height can be measured once a child is able to stand. Weight for length can then be plotted. For children older than 3, weight for age and height for age can be measured and plotted. Body mass index can then be calculated and plotted. Skin folds may be helpful but are not often routinely done as part of well child visits to the pediatrician. The National Center for Health Statistics (NCHS) through the Centers for Disease Control (CDC) and the World Health Organization have growth charts available for use.

20. D: The Mini Nutritional Assessment (MNA) is a nutrition tool that has been validated for use in the over age 65 population. The purpose of this tool is to screen for malnutrition or to identify those that may be at risk for developing malnutrition. The tool offers two different questionnaires. The first is a quick version that can be administered in about 3 minutes. The second is a more detailed questionnaire, which takes about 15 minutes and must be used if the short form indicates risk for malnutrition. Anyone can administer this tool and specialized training is not required. Health care professionals, such as dietitians, nurses, doctors, and others, can utilize this tool in a variety of settings.

21. B: The nutrition diagnosis is part of the nutrition care process. This is the step where the nutritional issue is identified and labeled using standardized language. A nutrition diagnosis is not made by a physician but rather an RD or a DTR depending upon the scope of practice. The nutrition diagnosis is organized and documented using a format of problem followed by etiology then signs and symptoms (PES). A standardized list is available for labeling the nutritional problem. An example of a PES is: Increased fat intake related to excessive consumption of fast food as evidenced by fasting serum cholesterol of 340 mg/dL. This statement leads the way for the nutrition intervention to be determined and implemented.

22. D: There are many, many potential nutrition diagnostic terminologies to select from for an obese male with coronary heart disease. The exact selection of the nutrition diagnosis would depend on the individual's diet history as well as other information. One potential may be related to caloric intake, such as excessive energy intake or imbalance of nutrients. Excessive hunger may be true but it is not considered proper terminology. Another potential nutrition diagnosis could be related to fat intake, such as excessive fat intake or inappropriate intake of food fats. Physical inactivity or inability or lack of desire to manage self-care may be potential choices depending upon the individual's exercise habits. Another potential can be in the biochemical category, such as altered nutrition related laboratory values (for example, an elevated serum cholesterol or triglyceride level). No one selection is wrong but rather how the issues are addressed and managed are incorrect.

23. C: There is a distinction between a nutrition diagnosis and a medical diagnosis. Type 1 diabetes mellitus, gestational diabetes, and hyperglycemia are all examples of medical diagnoses. A medical diagnosis will include disorders involving anatomy, physiology, or metabolism that have accompanying symptoms, which can be treated with either medical or surgical interventions. A patient with an elevated fasting blood glucose should also receive a nutrition diagnosis such as altered nutrition related laboratory value, excessive carbohydrate intake, excessive energy intake, or overweight/obesity. The nutrition diagnosis selected is dependent upon the information gathered by the RD or DTR during the assessment piece.

24. A: During pregnancy, the recommended amount of weight gain for a woman of normal weight is 25-35 pounds. For overweight women, a lower amount of weight gain, 15-25 lbs, is advised. Alternatively, underweight women are advised to gain 25-35 pounds. Typically, for a normal amount of weight gain, less than half of this consists of the fetus, the placenta, and the amniotic fluid. The additional weight is necessary to build-up maternal stores for the last part of the pregnancy and to help support lactation.

25. B: Folic acid is an extremely important vitamin for women of childbearing years. Adequate intake of folic acid reduces the incidence of neural tube defects (NTD), such as spina bifida. The requirements for folic acid increase during pregnancy from 400 µg to 600 µg. The neural tube closes by the 28th day of pregnancy. Many women do not even realize they are pregnant by this time; therefore, it is recommended that all women of childbearing age increase their folic acid intake to help prevent NTD. Other reasons for the increase in folic acid requirements are because of the expanding blood volume as well as growth of the fetus and the placenta.

26. C: Breastfeeding is highly recommended for all infants. If a woman chooses not to breastfeed, standard cow's milk formula at 20 cal/oz constitution can be offered. Breastfeeding infants should be allowed to breastfeed until they are satiated. The same is true for formula-fed infants. Force feeding a set amount of formula may lead to overfeeding and excessive weight gain. Adding rice cereal prior to 4-6 months of age is also not recommended. Adding rice cereal to the bottle at night may lead to excessive calorie intake and has not been definitely demonstrated to help infants sleep better. Weight gain should be carefully monitored to ensure that adequate calories are being consumed, and diapers should be monitored for adequate urine and stool output.

27. A: Preschool age is a time of rapid development in many areas including motor, cognitive, and social skills. Growth typically slows down during this period, and children often have a lower appetite. Children are also many times less interested in food because they are too interested in what is going on around them. Many develop picky eating habits, control issues over food, or even a very limited food preference list. Parents or caregivers should not force a child to eat. It won't work. Rather, a variety of foods should be offered on a fairly regular schedule. Preschoolers tend to consume what they need over the course of a day. Portion sizes do not have to be huge. Snacks should not be given less than 90 minutes before a meal. Beverages should also be restricted in the time before meals as this can reduce intake. Excessive juice should also be discouraged.

28. D: Metabolic syndrome is a compilation of multiple disorders, including insulin resistance, elevated glucose levels, hypertension, and elevated lipid levels. These disorders are dangerous alone and when linked together will increase the risk for Type 2 diabetes mellitus, heart disease, and stroke. Specific criteria have been developed in order to help diagnose the condition; fat in the abdominal area (known as apple shape) and insulin resistance are the most important indicators. Glucose levels higher than 110 mg/dL, triglycerides higher than 150 mg/dL, and HDL levels lower than 40 mg/dL in men and 50 mg/dL in women are all risk factors. A blood pressure reading greater than or equal to 135/85 mm Hg is a risk factor. Waist circumference measurements greater than 102 cm in men and 88 cm in women are risk factors. It is important to identify metabolic syndrome and to treat accordingly to reduce the chance of developing diabetes.

29. B: Initial treatment for metabolic syndrome includes lifestyle changes, such as diet and exercise habits, weight loss, and smoking cessation. A 5-10% initial weight loss is recommended with a longer-term goal of lowering BMI to less than 25 kg/m². Increasing physical activity to at least 30 min/day of moderate intensity most days of the week is also a goal. The TLC (Therapeutic Lifestyle Changes) diet should be implemented as a way to improve eating habits. This aims for reducing saturated fat intake to less than 7% of total calories, total fat intake to 35% or less of total calories, and increasing the amount of soluble fiber in the diet. The DASH diet is another possibility. Smoking cessation is also highly recommended. Medications may need to be added to lower lipid levels but may not be the initial therapy.

30. A: Celiac disease is a digestive disease involving the small intestine. The small intestine becomes damaged when any form of gluten is ingested. Symptoms may include diarrhea or constipation, change in appetite, nausea, excessive flatulence, or weight loss. Treatment is the implementation of a gluten-free diet. Some people may experience lactose intolerance prior to the celiac diagnosis but this often resolves once the gut begins to heal. Gluten is found in wheat, barley, rye, and bulgur. Typically, oats are also avoided though controversy remains about this. Corn, rice, and soy are acceptable grain products. Label reading is essential as many foods contain grain products. The selection of gluten-free products is growing making this a more manageable way of eating.

31. D: Diverticulitis is defined as an inflammation of an abnormal pouch-like sac in the wall of the intestine. Diverticulosis is the condition of having the pouch present. When the pouch or sac becomes inflamed, a low fiber (also referred to as low residue) diet should be initiated. This often begins with liquids. A diet high in fat may exacerbate the condition and a low-fat diet is usually better tolerated. The diet should be maintained until the inflammation subsides, and then fiber can be gradually added back into the diet. Tolerance should be monitored as fiber is being added. Once the individual is eating a normal diet, fiber intake should be maintained as high as possible with a goal of 30 g/ day. Adequate fluid and exercise are essential to keep the bowels working well and to prevent constipation. Nuts and seeds may be avoided if these foods have caused diverticulitis in the past.

32. B: Protein remains a very controversial nutrient for individuals with liver disease. For a patient with cirrhosis but without encephalopathy, the recommended protein intake is 0.8-1 g/kg to maintain positive nitrogen balance. The patient's estimated dry weight should be used for calculations. For a patient who is in negative nitrogen balance with cirrhosis without encephalopathy, this patient may need 1.2-1.3 g/kg. If this same patient is stressed, they may need as much as 1.5 g of protein per kg. The decision to restrict protein during acute encephalopathy is still unresolved. It is also imperative that adequate caloric intake be maintained.

33. C: There have been so many advances in the fields of diabetes and insulin regulation that the priority for any newly diagnosed patient should be to establish a meal plan first. The patient's usual eating habits, timing of meals, and food preferences need to be incorporated into the treatment plan. Once this is determined, the insulin regimen can be coordinated accordingly. Unfortunately, this does not always happen and patients are left to make drastic changes to their lifestyle to accommodate the insulin schedule. Weight loss is not always indicated for these patients, especially at the time of diagnosis. If weight loss is necessary, it is something that can be explored once the patient is metabolically stable. An insulin pump may indeed be an option for many patients but the meal plan is still first step.

34. D: Chromium supplementation has not yet been proven an effective means of lowering blood glucose levels for individuals with Type 2 diabetes mellitus. The most effective interventions are weight loss, physical activity, and reducing calorie intake. Weight loss helps improve insulin resistance. Even small amounts of weight loss can be beneficial, especially if weight is lost in the abdominal area. Increasing physical activity helps to lower blood glucose levels by making cells process glucose more effectively. It also helps with weight reduction. Reducing calorie intake has also been shown to be helpful in reducing blood glucose levels.

35. A: Alcohol may be permitted if the following conditions are met: diabetes and blood glucose are well controlled, diabetic nerve damage is not present, and the person has a good understanding of how alcohol affects diabetes. Alcohol should be limited to 1 drink per day for women, which is equivalent to 5 oz of wine or 12 oz of beer. For men, the limit is 2 drinks per day. Alcohol should never be taken on an empty stomach as it increases the risk for hypoglycemia. Additionally, alcohol should never be substituted for food. Alcohol is metabolized in the liver, and the liver will temporarily stop blood glucose regulation until the alcohol is cleared. This means that if the blood glucose level is low; it has a good chance of dropping even lower and potentially causing problems.

36. C: There are approximately 90 g of carbohydrate in the described breakfast. 4 oz of juice and ½ of a banana contribute approximately 15 g each. One slice of bread and ½ cup of oatmeal each contribute 15 g. One tablespoon of jelly contributes approximately 15 g as well. Reading food labels is one way to know how many carbohydrates are in certain foods. This method of keeping track of carbohydrate intake is called carbohydrate counting. It is a way for people to know how many grams of carbohydrates they are eating and how this affects blood glucose levels. Fine tuning the total amount of carbohydrates at each meal and snack is important for good control.

37. B: There are a number of risk factors for developing cardiovascular disease (CVD). Category I risk factors are risk factors that have been definitively proven to reduce overall risk through intervention. These risk factors include smoking cessation, lowering LDL cholesterol, reducing blood pressure, treating thrombogenic issues, and diet modification for fat and cholesterol. Conversely, there are risk factors that will never be able to be modified, such as age, male gender, and family history of early CVD. Low socioeconomic status is another risk factor that is difficult to modify. These are considered Category IV risk factors. Category II risk factors, such as diabetes, lack of physical activity, HDL level, and obesity, will likely improve CVD risk if these risk factors are addressed. Category III risk factors may possibly lower CVD risk if intervention is provided. These risk factors include improving homocysteine level, reducing alcohol intake, and improving psychosocial situation.

38. B: The 2 main omega-3-fatty acids are eicosapentaenoic acid (EPA) and docosahexaenoic acid (DHA). These are found primarily in fish sources, such as fish oil and fish from the ocean. Omega3-fatty acids along with omega-6-fatty acids are essential fatty acids. These fatty acids cannot be made by the body and therefore must be supplied through diet. Omega-3-fatty acids can help lower triglyceride levels and are thought to reduce overall CVD risk. Omega-3-fatty acids also help reduce the rate of atherosclerotic plaque that accumulates in the arteries. To ensure adequate intake of essential fatty acids, it is recommended that fatty fish be consumed at least twice per week or other sources of fatty acids, such as flaxseed, canola, and soybean oils as well as walnuts and flaxseed be included in the diet.

39. D: Trans fatty acids are created through the hydrogenation process that is used to prevent polyunsaturated fats from spoiling. It also helps liquid oil retain a solid form. Trans fats are thought to increase the risk of cardiovascular disease (CVD). They also increase LDL cholesterol levels, lower HDL cholesterol levels, and increase overall cholesterol. Trans fats also cause inflammation of vessels and are linked to obesity and insulin resistance. Trans fats are mostly found in fried foods, baked goods, processed foods, and some margarines. The food industry is taking major steps to eliminate trans fats from many products. Food labeling requirements now mandate that the amount of trans fat be included on all food labels. The restaurant industry is also taking steps to reduce trans-fat and hydrogenated oil usage although not all restaurants or fast food chains are presently working toward this goal.

40. A: Soluble fiber has been shown to help lower blood cholesterol levels. Foods that contain soluble fiber include oat bran and oatmeal, dried beans and peas, rice bran, citrus fruit, strawberries, and apples. Commercially prepared products such as oat bran muffins may actually contain very little fiber and may also contain trans fatty acids; therefore, these foods are not recommended. Insoluble fiber does not appear to lower blood cholesterol levels but has other benefits, such as normalizing bowel function. Foods that contain insoluble fiber include whole wheat breads and cereals, wheat bran, carrots, Brussels sprouts, and cauliflower. A total of 25-30 g of fiber should be consumed each day with at least 6-10 g from soluble fiber sources.

41. C: The National Cholesterol Education Program (NCEP) devised a diet called the Therapeutic Lifestyle Changes diet (TLC) as part of the Expert Panel on Detection, Evaluation, and Treatment of High Blood Cholesterol in Adults (ATP III panel). This diet serves to replace the old Step I and II diet. The diet is geared for people who are at high risk for cardiovascular disease (CVD) or already have CVD. The diet consists of sufficient calories to achieve or maintain a healthy body weight; total fat intake limited to 25-35% of total calories, with less than 7% from saturated sources; cholesterol intake less than 200 mg/day; and 2400 mg or less of sodium per day. Additionally, it is recommended that complex sources of carbohydrates be included as well as 10-25 g soluble fiber and 2 g/day of a plant sterol or stanol.

42. D: For individuals who wish to initiate aggressive dietary intervention in an effort to avoid medication or to more aggressively try to achieve blood lipid goals while receiving cholesterol lowering medications, a very low-fat diet may be tried. This is not a popular option nor is it an easy plan to follow. This type of diet is basically a vegetarian option although egg whites and nonfat dairy products are allowed. All meat, fish, and poultry are omitted. Other protein sources include soy products and dried beans and legumes. The rest of the diet consists of whole grain products, fruits, and vegetables. Added fats in the form of oils or margarine are not allowed. Foods that contain good types of fat, such as nuts or seeds, are also omitted.

43. C: One purpose of nutrition screening is to identify risk factors that have been associated with nutritional issues. Nutrition screen also helps to identify malnourished individuals in a timelier manner. The process allows individuals to be more efficiently and quickly identified so nutrition intervention can be initiated. Known risk factors for malnutrition or risk factors that may increase the risk of developing malnutrition are useful in this process. Once an individual is identified in the screening process, a full nutrition assessment can be completed and nutrition care initiated. Body mass index may be utilized in the screening process though this is not generally the purpose of the screen.

44. B: There are many lifestyle changes that can be made to promote lower hypertension, but the most beneficial change is weight loss. Research shows that the risk for developing hypertension is up to 6 times higher in people who are overweight. As much as a third of all cases of hypertension are due to being overweight. The Framingham Heart Study has shown that a 10% gain in weight can lead to an increase of 7 mm Hg in blood pressure. The dangers of hypertension include damage to kidney function, changes in insulin resistance, and hyperinsulinemia. Losing weight leads to a lower vascular resistance, reduces total blood volume thus reducing the amount of effort needed to pump blood, and lower cardiac output as well as improvement in insulin resistance. Even a 5% reduction in weight provides almost immediate benefits.

45. A: With overweight and obesity rising in this country, the incidence of hypertension is also rising. It is important for children to have yearly blood pressure checks to monitor for hypertension. Primary hypertension does occur and many times is due to weight. If a child's BMI is above 30, intensive nutrition education is recommended. The overall goal for educating adolescents with hypertension or at risk for developing hypertension is to address lifestyle issues that will impact the child for many, many years. These issues include weight control, reducing sodium intake, and increasing physical activity.

46. D: The DASH diet stands for Dietary Approaches to Stop Hypertension. Studies were done by the National Heart, Lung, and Blood Institute (NHLBI) that demonstrated a reduction in blood pressure in response to a diet that was low in total fat and saturated fat, low in cholesterol and sodium, and also included foods that were high in other nutrients, such as magnesium, potassium, and calcium. The general DASH diet nutrient guidelines are: limited total calories from fat to 27%, with up to 6% coming from saturated sources; 150 mg cholesterol; 18% of total calories from protein; and 55% of total calories from carbohydrates. For 1800 calories, this would equal 55 g of fat (495 calories) with 12 g of saturated fat, 80 g of protein (320 calories), and 250 g of carbohydrate (1000 calories). The guidelines also call for 2300 mg of sodium per day with an option of 1500 mg, and 30 g of fiber.

47. C: Higher potassium intake has been linked to lower blood pressure readings. Increasing potassium intake has also been linked to a reduced risk for strokes. The DASH diet recommends approximately 90 mEq of potassium each day. Good sources of potassium include vegetables, such as potatoes, sweet potatoes, spinach, tomatoes, and squash; as well as fruits, such as bananas, apricots, oranges, and cantaloupe. Legumes, such as soybeans, lentils, kidney beans, and split peas, are also a rich source of potassium. Nuts, such as almonds and walnuts, can also contribute significant amounts of potassium. Dairy products, such as milk and yogurt, as well as protein choices, such as pork and beef, are also good sources.

48. A: Individuals with congestive heart failure (CHF) should try to limit their sodium intake to less than 3000 mg/day and ideally 2000 mg/day. Too much sodium causes fluid retention, and this extra fluid puts an additional strain on the heart. It can cause difficulty breathing (dues to aspiration) as well as swelling of different body parts, =such as the legs or ankles. Furthermore, with Lasix use, adequate potassium is essential because Lasix causes the body to excrete potassium as it works to get rid of excess fluid. Fluids are often restricted for people with CHF. Fluids are typically limited to 500-2000 ml/day while in the hospital. At home, fluid intake is more liberal if the CHF is under good control. Monitoring weight in the morning is recommended.

49. B: A high protein diet is more appropriate in the immediate post-transplant period due to stress of surgery, catabolism due to high dose steroids, and the need for wound healing. As the patient recovers and the steroids are weaned, the need for a high protein diet is not usually warranted. The main nutritional concerns post-transplant address side effects of the immunosuppressive medication. Glucose intolerance is a common side effect of many medications. Many of the medications also cause weight gain or increased appetite. Cholesterol management is also extremely important as many long-term transplant survivors will experience atherosclerosis of the graft, which may ultimately lead to death. Other potential long-term complications of transplants include hypertension and osteopenia.

50. C: Patients with chronic obstructive pulmonary disease (COPD) are at high risk for malnutrition due to a number of factors. Poor respiratory function can negatively impact appetite, food intake, one's ability to prepare food, and increase caloric requirement with the increased effort to breathe. The prognosis for individuals who develop malnutrition is not as favorable as for those without malnutrition. Nutrition intervention is usually geared towards ensuring adequate caloric, protein, vitamin, and mineral intake as well as providing a balanced diet, which prevents carbon dioxide retention. Overall outcome measures for this population include improvements in weight status and nutritional status. Outcome measures may also include improvements in ADLs, such as meal preparation. Outcomes correlating with renal function are not necessarily measured unless renal dysfunction was preexisting.

51. B: The National Kidney Foundation's Kidney Dialysis Outcome Quality Initiative (KDOQI) developed nutritional recommendations for individuals with ESRD. For those with a glomerular function less than 25 ml/min and who have not started any form of dialysis, a limit of 0.6 g/kg of protein is suggested. It is very important to adjust caloric intake such that protein is spared from being used as calories. Thus, for the aforementioned patients, 35 kcal/kg, daily, is recommended. About half of the protein intake should come from high biological value. The amount of protein being consumed should be adjusted based on renal function, nutritional status, and ability to consume adequate calories.

52. A: Use the American Dietetic Association's Exchange List for Meal Planning as a reference. The diet recall shows the patient consumed approximately 108 g of protein. This provided her with 1.8 g/kg. Protein requirements for continuous ambulatory peritoneal dialysis (CAPD) are approximately 1.2-1.3 g/kg. The laboratory data does not indicate that the woman requires additional protein for repletion of visceral stores. This woman could safely reduce her protein intake to the recommended range by reducing portion sizes of protein containing foods, such as chicken or milk. Care should be taken to ensure she is consuming sufficient calories (30-35 kcal/kg) for weight maintenance.

53. C: Mucositis is defined as inflammation of the mucous membranes usually in the mouth, but it can also occur along the digestive tract. The consistency of a patient's diet can be altered to alleviate some of the pain from mucositis. Examples of diet modification include soft, bland foods void of extremes in temperatures. Avoidance of salty, sour, citrus, and spicy foods and alcohol is generally recommended. Xerostomia is defined as abnormal dryness of the mouth. This side effect can be addressed by avoiding tobacco and alcohol and adequately hydrating. Soft, moist foods are recommended; foods that stick to the roof of the mouth should be limited. Sugarless candies, gum, and lemon may stimulate the flow of saliva.

54. D: Many interventions may be employed to encourage a child to eat greater quantities. Small meals and snacks should be offered throughout the day to try to gradually increase the amount of food a child is eating. A variety of foods should be offered. When the child feels hungry, it is important to capitalize on this moment and offer a larger meal. Limiting the amount of fluid the child drinks with meals is important so the child does not feel too full from liquid calories. Presenting the food in an interesting way, such as in different shapes or on fun plates, may encourage the child to eat more. Increasing physical activity may also stimulate the child's appetite.

55. C: The National Dysphagia Diet (NDD) was published in 2002 by the American Dietetic Association as a method to streamline the language and definitions used for texture modified diets. The NDD involved a panel of experts including dietitians, speech language pathologists, and a food scientist. There are 4 levels to the diet ranging from Level 1 to regular consistency. Level 1 is a dysphagia pureed diet where food is cohesive and does not need to be formed into a bolus. Minimal chewing ability is required. Level 2 is dysphagia- mechanical altered consistency, which means that the food is moist and semisolid requiring just a little chewing. Level 3 is dysphagia advanced, which is a soft diet that does require some chewing skills. Last is the regular level, in which there are no texture restrictions. The NDD also provides specific terms for liquids including thin, nectar-like, honey-like, and spoon thick.

56. B: Healthy People 2030 is a program administered through the Department of Health and Human Services that aims to address health issues within our nation and help reduce the impact of these issues. The overall goals are to help individuals live longer and to have a better quality of life. Another goal is to try to eradicate differences in health between different population groups. There are a number of leading health indicators that are utilized to determine if the overall health of the nation is improving. It also includes 62 focus areas, such as diabetes, cancer, food safety, heart disease, and health education to help organizations determine what areas to target.

57. A: The Dietary Reference Intake (DRI) was initiated in 1997 by the Institute of Medicine as part of the US National Academy of Sciences. It is used for many purposes including menu development. The DRIs incorporate the Recommended Dietary Allowances (RDA), Adequate Intake (AI), Tolerable Upper Limits (TUL), and Estimated Average Requirements (EAR). The RDAs were developed from the EAR values. The EAR values are appropriate for most people. The AI values are used for nutrients where no RDA has been determined but the value selected is believed to be safe. The TUL values should be heeded as levels of certain nutrients in amounts higher than the TUL may be harmful All the items listed are important to consider when menu planning.

58. C: The 2005 Dietary Guidelines for Americans incorporated evidence-based recommendations in 9 topic areas. The 2000 guidelines recommended plenty of fruits, vegetables, and whole grains; however, the 2005 guidelines provide recommendations to consume vegetables from specific color categories, such as 3 cups/week of dark green and 2 cups/week of orange vegetables. These guidelines also provide specific guidelines for consuming 3 servings/day of breads, cereals, or pasta with the remainder from whole grain products. The guidelines also recommend achieving and maintaining a healthy body weight and engaging in at least 60 minutes of moderate activity most days of the week. Other recommendations include minimizing fat intake to no more than 20-35% of total calories and saturated fat to less than 10% of total calories; consuming 3 servings/day of dairy and less than 2300 mg of sodium per day; and limiting alcohol intake to one drink/day for women and 2 for men. The guidelines also address food safety.

59. D: Generally, a fractured femur does not present nutritional risk unless other risk factors are also present. Physical conditions presenting nutritional risk include obesity, severely underweight, or an unplanned weight loss of more than 10 pounds over a 6-month period. Pregnant adolescents, multiple gestation, or women who have had multiple pregnancies in a very short time would also be considered at nutritional risk. Certain diseases, such as diabetes, cardiac and kidney disorders, may increase a person's risk. Individuals with cancer or AIDS are at nutritional risk. Altered skin integrity, such as decubitus ulcers or burns, are nutritional risk factors as well.

60. D: A DTR can work at a long-term care facility under the direction of an RD. Visiting patients during meals is one function a DTR may perform. The DTR can perform visual observation of a patient's progress with meals. A DTR can visually assess whether an individual is consuming a certain percentage of meals, and this information is helpful in making additional recommendations for nutritional care. The DTR can visually observe whether someone is having difficulty with utensil use and may benefit from the services of an occupational therapist. The DTR can also observe whether the patient is consuming the supplements ordered for them or assist with finding an alternative. Making dietary texture recommendations for and observations of a patient who has had a stroke is difficult as medications may be necessary to accommodate swallowing, not chewing, issues.

61. A: There are many types of documentation styles but the ADIME style is the one that was developed to help facilitate the NCP. ADIME stands for <u>A</u>ssessment, <u>D</u>iagnosis, <u>I</u>ntervention, <u>M</u>onitoring, and <u>E</u>valuation. This type of charting format helps to organize the information in the appropriate manner. Nutrition professionals are moving away from the SOAP format because notes tend to be lengthy; physicians do not appear to be as receptive to this type of charting; and it takes away from the evaluation or assessment piece, which is what DTRs and RDs are the most qualified to contribute. The ADIME format incorporates all important information necessary to make the assessment and the PES statement to make the nutrition diagnosis. It also includes the intervention piece, such as change in nutrient intake, nutrition education, counseling, or the coordination of nutrition care. The data to be monitored and evaluated is also charted, such as changes in weight, laboratory values, or improvement in clinical symptoms.

62. D: The pancreas is an important organ in the digestive process. It has both endocrine functions (secretion of insulin and glucagon for blood glucose) and exocrine functions (secretion of pancreatic enzymes to help with digestion of fat, protein, and carbohydrate). As food enters the stomach, secretion of pancreatic enzymes occurs. If an individual has either acute or chronic pancreatitis, food is withheld until the condition subsides to prevent this secretion. Some pancreatic tumors may be cured if detected early; however, most cases with this type of tumor are not found early, which negatively impacts prognosis. Tumors that are in the head of the pancreas are most likely to respond to curative treatment.

63. B: The Supplemental Nutrition Assistance Program (SNAP) was formerly called the Food Stamp program. It is a federally funded program administered by the United States Department of Agriculture's Food and Nutrition Service. Congress passed the last law in 2008, called the Food, Conservation and Energy Act of 2008 as part of the Farm Bill. Income eligibility is no more than 130% of the poverty level for gross monthly income or 100% of the poverty level for net monthly income. Adjustments have been made to the law to enable consumers to have a certain amount of money in the bank and other assets, such as a car or a house worth a certain amount. Retirement and education accounts are not counted. Children who receive SNAP benefits are automatically eligible for free school breakfast and lunch programs. There are also employment requirements as well as rules for the elderly and disabled.

64. D: Federal requirements mandate that specific foods be available to those participating in the WIC program. All WIC foods must meet the Food and Drug Administration's Standards of Identity to qualify. Breakfast cereals have iron requirements and sucrose limitations. Breads must be whole grain and contain a certain percentage of whole grains. Juice must be 100% juice and not flavored drinks. Most types of milk are acceptable, including flavored and soy. Cheese is also included as long as is not a processed spread or imported. Yogurt is not an option. Tofu, eggs, peanut butter, most legumes, and canned fish are all available protein choices. Most fruits and vegetables in the fresh, frozen or canned forms are acceptable, however, white potatoes, condiments, salad bar items, and fruit roll up type products are not allowed. There are also many infant products available, such as infant cereal and jarred foods; however, packages for lactating moms will vary if formula is being supplemented.

65. A: The Stages of Change model (also known as the transtheoretical model) describes 6 phases associated with readiness to make a change. It is helpful for nutrition professionals to assess an individual's stage of change when initiating education about diet changes. The individual described in the question is in the contemplative stage. The individual knows that weight loss is necessary but has not yet taken the steps to enter the action phase where successful weight loss should occur. Providing excuses and reasons for not being successful is an indication that the individual is still only thinking about the changes needed to achieve weight loss. It is here that the educator should help the individual look at advantages and disadvantages to help them move towards the preparation and action phases.

66. C: This client is displaying resistant behavior. This type of behavior can be observed in many different ways, such as frequent interruption and offering excuses. Also, a client may try to tell you what is wrong with your suggestions for making change by saying "Yes, but…" Some clients will remain in denial about needing to change or will try to blame another person for being unable to follow nutrition advice. The client may also question the professional's ability to educate or their knowledge on the subject being discussed. A client with resistant behavior may also be very hostile.

67. D: When an individual is ready to make changes, it is imperative to get the individual involved in making the plan. The job of the RD or DTR is not to tell the client what to do but instead help the individual identify areas where changes can be made. Options can be provided but ultimately it is the individual who must decide what changes to make. The RD or DTR can help the individual set short term goals. Any potential barriers should be identified and discussed. The client should be able to verbalize the plan on his or her own but a written plan should also be given. The main point is for the individual, not the counselor, to be in control of the plan.

68. D: Motivations interviewing is a direct and patient-centered method for dietetic practitioners to counsel a patient. The practitioner should express empathy and encouragement while using reflective listening techniques. Reflective listening entails listening to what the patient is saying then making a statement interpreting how the patient feels. The counselor needs to continuously determine the patient's state of readiness for change in order to prevent resistance. The patient is allowed freedom to make his or her own choices assuming that motivation is internal and will be sufficient to provide motivation from within. The counselor does not judge the patient or confront him or her. The patient talks more than the counselor. This style works best if a patient is ambivalent or not ready to change their diet because it helps them to explore the reasons for this.

69. B: Self-monitoring is a technique used in nutrition counseling that has had evidence of improved outcomes. This technique utilizes record keeping of any behavior that may negatively or positively impact food choices or weight. An example of recorded data includes the amount of food, time, and place food was eaten. Specific nutrients may be recorded, such as carbohydrates or fat. Another example is recording any type of emotion that is felt when eating or any negativism in terms of body image or success. Clinical data includes weight, blood pressure, or blood glucose. Successes should be enjoyed and celebrated. Feedback should be provided to help the client fine tune what he or she is recording.

70. B: On-the-job training is a type of training that is usually completed on-site and typically has good results. It helps develop good working relationships with other employees and supervisors, helps people feel a sense of accomplishment that they have learned the appropriate skills required to do the job, and helps reduce costs by protecting equipment from accidental breakage due to knowledge deficit. Generally, the one who is training tries to make the employee comfortable in order to learn. The trainer shows the employee how to complete each task and emphasizes key issues. The employee should then be able to demonstrate tasks and be able to verbally explain them as well. Follow up is important to ensure complete and adequate training as well as to answer remaining questions.

71. A: Diversity training is not limited to race and gender topics; rather it encompasses age, sexual orientation, degree of seniority on the job, different types of jobs, etc. Diversity training is necessary even if the work group appears to be similar in appearance, belief, abilities, etc. Individuals within the group are different and free thinking. Diversity sensitivity should be an integral part of an organization's culture. Communication should always be open and any conflicts should be addressed directly. Interpersonal skills are also an important part of diversity training. It should be the expectation that each employee treats one another with respect and support. A workplace should never be hostile, and the employees that work there should be thoroughly trained to deal with differences.

72. A: An icebreaker encourages individuals taking part in a meeting to participate, listen to others, and allows for fun and/or interesting dialog. Typically, icebreakers are used to begin a meeting. Icebreakers are also used to gauge the participants' current level of knowledge regarding the topic at hand. Some icebreakers are also team building exercises. Icebreakers are often useful when they are directly related to the topic of the training session and/or are used to increase interest in future trainings.

73. C: Effective nutrition education encompasses many factors. Educational information should be presented in a clear, concise manner but with repetition to emphasize important points. It is also important to let the audience know in advance what you will be discussing by using words such as first, second, or next. The use of plain language is recommended because it helps to reach a wider range of people with varying literacy levels. Approximately half of the population reads at a reading level somewhere between the 5th and 8th grade. Many of these people will not understand and comprehend information presented to them at a reading level higher than that. Use plain language to simplify and visual aids to clarify presented information.

74. D: A selective menu is a menu that gives at least two choices in each of the categories listed on the menu, such as appetizers, salads, entrees, vegetables or sides, desserts, and beverages. A semi-selective menu offers at least one choice in a few of the menu categories but not all. For example, at certain health care facilities, a choice of two entrees and two desserts may be offered but soup and vegetable choices are not offered. A static menu is a menu where the same choices are offered each day. Occasionally the choices may include specials to increase variety. A nonselective menu is also referred to as a preselected menu and does not offer choices in any of the categories. Typically, a list of alternatives or substitutes is available for those who do not like the choices, and these are written in on the menu.

75. A: A cycle menu is a menu that is planned to cover a certain number of days or weeks on a rotating schedule. The length of the cycle is determined by the institution utilizing the cycle menu. Many hospitals are now trying shorter cycles because of decreased lengths of stay. Other types of facilities, such as nursing homes, have longer cycles. Cycle menus do facilitate schedules because the menu is known in advance.

Equipment use can be maximized with cycle menus because recipes are chosen in advance and with consideration of equipment availability. Variety, however, is not always an advantage of cycle menus because the cycle may be too short or repeated in a very predictable manner, such as on the same day of each week.

76. C: Menu planning involves thinking about and visualizing how the food will look on the plate when served. In the example, the food is monochrome and not visually pleasing. Color is important in menus and at least two different color items should be offered at a meal. There are so many different types and colors of vegetables that it should never be problematic to find one that is in season and affordable to add to a menu. Other menu characteristics to consider include texture, consistency, and shapes. Varying flavors is also important as too many strong flavors may not go well together. Varying the method of food preparation is also important.

77. D: It is important for food service operations that operate in healthcare facilities to utilize the services of nutrition professionals in order to comply with written physician diet orders. The master menu and diet manual are necessary in order to create modified menu extenders. This collaboration ensures the master menu can also meet the needs of those requiring special diets. For example, if baked chicken is planned for regular diets, the entrée must be evaluated for different texture consistencies, sodium, and/or fat modifications and appropriateness or for individuals with diabetes. This ensures that the meal is in compliance with the written diet order and that appropriate foods are being served to the residents of the facility. It also helps the purchasing process as any special foods will are identified.

78. B: A spoken menu is used in many healthcare facilities due to the shorter lengths of stays. A spoken menu enables more personalized service and this usually equates with improved customer satisfaction. Because the lengths of stay are now shorter, an extensive menu is not usually required because most patients do not stay long enough to feel bored with the menu. A spoken menu also allows costs to be reduced because paper and printing costs are eliminated. The process of planning the menu is simpler because it takes less time to process the menu and it can be easily adapted to food that is in season.

79. C: Determining customer satisfaction is a very important part of the menu planning process. It is a subjective process that involves interpreting opinions, perspectives, and perceptions of the menu. There are a few tools that can be used to determine customer satisfaction. Comment cards and surveys may be used and include any number of questions regarding the food. These may include inquiries regarding portion sizes, overall taste and appearance, service provided, and tray accuracy. Surveys can be done in house or after discharge. Observational studies and plate waste studies are other ways to gauge customer satisfaction. Eavesdropping is not the best choice but informal comments can be obtained from listening to customers talk. Customer perception is an important element when determining satisfaction.

80. C: Food purchased within a state and shipped intrastate is subject to regulations enforced by the US Department of Agriculture, which is responsible for the regulation of meat, poultry, and other types of processed foods. It is also subject to regulation by the Food and Drug Administration, which is responsible for enforcing the production, manufacturing, distribution, and labeling of many food items with the exception of meat, eggs, and poultry. All state and local regulations, which are equal to or greater than federal regulations, must also be followed. In some cases, the regulations are more stringent. The Food and Nutrition Service, as part of the USDA, deals mainly with hunger assistance, not food regulation.

81. B: The Food and Drug Association manages many of the laws and regulations pertaining to food. The Food and Drug Cosmetic Act, 1938, is responsible for establishing standards of identity that specify ingredient requirements for food classification. There are standards of identity for many food products, including chocolate, ice cream, milk, and others. Other standards include the standard of quality, which specifies both quality of ingredients and acceptable defects; and standards of fill, which specifies the ingredient amount in a product (designed to prevent consumer deception). For example, a can of vegetables must contain a standard amount of vegetable and water dependent upon can size.

82. C: Although a Web site is a very important tool for any company, it is not necessarily one of the most important points in vendor selection. The relationship between a vendor and a food service operation is very important and merits careful consideration. The vendor is important to the overall functioning of the business or operation. A vendor should have acceptable policies regarding deliveries during emergencies and disasters; refunding and/or crediting the buyer if products are not satisfactory, and others. Recommendations from other food service providers are also helpful when evaluating a vendor's ability to meet contract specifications and deadlines. Value added services, such as service programs and provision of specialized equipment, are also important factors to consider when selecting a vendor.

83. D: There are eight potential grades for beef. Prime is the top of the line beef that is the most flavorful and tender. Choice is the second highest designation, and it has three different grade levels—small, modest, and moderate marbling. Moderate marbling in a choice cut is one step below prime and will yield a tasty and tender product. Select cut is the third designation; select cuts are tender but less tasty (due to less marbling) than higher designations. Prime, Choice and Select beef are available at supermarkets. The other cuts of beef are standard, commercial, utility, cutter, and canner with canner being the lowest quality. These cuts are used in commercially prepared products such as sausages, hot dogs, and other beef products.

84. A: The Agricultural Marketing Act of 1946 established a grading system for many agricultural products, including fruits and vegetables. The use of the grading system is voluntary. Meat, poultry, fresh fruits, and vegetables are typically labeled with this grading system. Processed fruits and vegetables do not typically utilize the grading process. The standard grades for processed fruits and vegetables are US Grade A, or Fancy; US Grade B, or Extra-Standard; US Grade C, or Standard; and Substandard. One way that manufacturers address quality issues is to develop private labels and build a consumer following. These products may not exactly correspond to the government's grading system, and there may be variations between seasons.

85. B: There are several different types of inventory systems in food service. One system is the par stock system. This system establishes a required minimum number for each product stock. For example, if the DTR in this case was using the par stock system and chose to order 1 case of peaches, the par level must be 2 because that would be the number on-hand after delivery. The min-max system of inventory set a maximum amount of product in stock at any one time. It also determines a minimum amount of product in stock, and when the inventory reaches this specific level, the product is replenished to the maximum level. In this example, the numbers do not add up to a maximum level. Although inventory does involve some degree of instinct and experience to order correctly, it is most often done in a systematic manner.

86. C: Receiving is a very important process. The receiving area should be located close to the delivery dock and near the storage area. This helps reduce the amount of traffic through the production area. The delivery should be checked by a well-trained employee to determine if the order matches the delivery as well as to inspect the quality of the deliverables. The delivery should be checked against the purchase order and should also be verified against the invoice as well. When receiving frozen goods, they should be inspected prior to moving into the freezer to ensure the products are still frozen and have not been thawed and refrozen during transport. All food should be checked for quality, and it is a good idea to randomly check cases or crates to verify contents. Security in the receiving area is important to prevent theft.

87. B: The dry storage area must be dry and well ventilated. The appropriate temperature for a dry storage area is between 50-70 degrees with humidity between 50-70% to prevent the growth of mold. Food placed 8 inches off the ground is appropriate. Flour or other types of food products should be stored in air tight containers once they have been opened. Inventory should be stored using the FIFO (first in, first out) approach. This ensures that older inventory is used before the newer products. New inventory should always be placed at the back. Paper products can be stored in the dry storage area but most health codes require that chemicals and cleaning supplies be stored in a different location for safety reasons.

88. D: A list of suggested maximum storage times and temperatures should be readily available to employees who monitor the inventory. Ground beef should be held at a temperature no higher than 38 degrees for no longer than 2 days. In the interest of food safety, this should be discarded. Hard cooked eggs, if refrigerated at a maximum temperature of 40 degrees, can be held for up to 7 days. Hard cheese that is wrapped tightly and held at a maximum temperature of 40 degrees is good for up to 6 months. Leftover beef stew held at a maximum temperature of 40 degrees is good for up to 4 days. Leafy vegetables that have not been washed can stay good up to 7 days, and root vegetables, such as potatoes and onions can be held for at least a month. Fruits can vary from a week to 2 weeks depending upon the kind of fruit.

89. B: Forecasting is the term used for predicting how much food is needed for specific period, such as a day or an event. Forecasting helps the purchasing area know what type of food to buy and how much is required. The production area needs this information to determine how much of an item is needed and where it will be served, such as tray line or cafeteria. Accurate forecasting can be difficult, but it is important to make the best possible prediction in order to prevent waste or loss of money. In smaller facilities, menu items for patients are often tallied, but in larger operations, different methods are used that involve information on historical data, census or number of students enrolled, other staff purchasing meals, and other information. Computers can also be utilized for this process. The weather also needs to be taken into account when making a forecast.

90. C: A standardized recipe is one that has been extensively tested in the facility where the recipe will be utilized to ensure it meets the needs of the facility. These needs may include factors such as customer satisfaction, use of equipment, or financial. It is considered a control tool. Standardized recipes help ensure the product is consistent in flavor and composition each time it is served Standardized recipes facilitate other areas of food service, such as production, purchasing, and centralized ingredient area. Food service systems that are computerized require standardized recipes to work as a trigger point of many different functions, such as developing the production schedule. It should include the title of the recipe, the yield and portion size, list of ingredients and amounts needed as well as how cooking time and temperature. If the chef is planning on extending the recipe, it should be adjusted ahead of time.

91. A: There are two methods that are frequently used to adjust the yield of recipes- the factor and percentage methods. The factor method involves dividing the desired yield by the actual yield, in this case 50/8. Next, all the measures are converted to weights then the amount each ingredient needed is multiplied by the factor. Fractions are then rounded off to a usable number. In the percentage method, each ingredient is measured as a percentage of the total weight of the product. The sum of the percentages of all ingredients should add up to 100. The percentage value is then used for further recipe adjustments.

92. C: A cook/hot-hold type of food service is one where food is prepared and heated to the desired final temperature then held hot on the tray line. Food is then portioned, and the trays are assembled. Trays are transported to the patient unit and delivered to the patient immediately. This is an example of a centralized system. A cook/freeze or cook/chill system involves an initial heating of the food product followed by either freezing or chilling then storage until needed. At that time, the products are heated to a final desired temperature. In a heat/serve system, commercially prepared foods are used and no initial heating is done.

93. D: The Americans with Disabilities Act (ADA), effective July of 1992, prohibits any discrimination against anyone who has a disability. It also guarantees equal opportunities for people with disabilities in two main areas--employment and public accommodations, such as transportation and facilities. When planning a hospital cafeteria renovation, it is imperative to follow the law exactly. The law requires reasonable accommodation to make facilities accessible to all people. There are checklists available to help with planning. The list includes items such as widening of doorways to accommodate wheelchairs, addition of ramps, lowering shelves, and adapting other workspaces. This law applies to all employers who have more than 15 employees, has federal contracts worth over $10,000, or receives federal financial assistance.

94. B: Food poisoning caused by staphylococcus aureus (staph aureus) is typically caused when the person serving food cross contaminates from other products. It can also be caused by equipment that has not been properly cleaned. Foods that are likely to cause this type of infection include egg products; salads, such as potato or tuna salad; and cream-type dessert foods, such as custard or cream puffs. Chicken and cooked meats can also cause this. The onset of symptoms is usually 1-6 hours and will last approximately 2 days. The symptoms include vomiting, diarrhea, nausea, lack of appetite, abdominal pain, and distention. This type of microorganism can be verified through a stool culture. It can live in the nasal passages and throats as well as on the hair and skin.

95. B: E. coli is a microorganism that lives within the intestines and is beneficial to health. Other types of E. coli such as E. coli 0157:H7 are very dangerous and can cause severe illness. This type of E. coli can be found in undercooked beef but especially in ground beef, raw fruits and vegetables, soft cheeses, unpasteurized dairy products, and contaminated water. The onset of this type of infection is between 1-8 days and can last as long as 10 days. The main symptom of E. coli infection is severe diarrhea that is often accompanied by blood. Vomiting and abdominal pain are also likely; however, fever is not usually present. This can also lead to hemolytic uremic syndrome, which leads to acute kidney failure. E. coli poisoning can be prevented by washing all foods including meats, fruits and vegetables thoroughly and cooking to the appropriate temperature.

96. D: Listeria is a type of bacteria that can be found in raw foods, processed foods, such as hot dogs and deli meats, as well as dairy products, such as soft cheeses. Listeria is unique in that it can grow in cooler temperatures including the refrigerator. Listeria is especially dangerous to pregnant women as it can lead to stillbirth or delivering prematurely. The symptoms of listeriosis include muscle aches, nausea, and diarrhea. The symptoms can be similar to those of the flu. Other high-risk groups include people with compromised immune systems. People older than 60 and infants are also at higher infection risk as they may suffer long-term brain damage from infection.

97. A: The danger zone is the temperature range between 41-140°F. This is the range where bacteria can multiply and grow to potentially cause illness. Freezing foods stops the growth of bacteria but does not necessarily kill the bacteria. Temperatures above 165°F will kill most bacteria. Situations that put food at risk for becoming contaminated include foods that are not properly cooled or heated, foods prepared a day or more in advance before they are served, and mixing contaminated raw ingredients into foods that will not be cooked further. Poor food service employee hygiene and equipment cleaning can increase the risk for infection. Basic prevention includes chilling food quickly to less than 41°F, storing cold foods at a temperature less than 41°F and hot foods at temperatures above 135°F.

98. C: The Health Insurance Portability and Accountability Act of 1996, is also known as HIPAA. Within HIPAA, there is a privacy rule called Standards for Privacy of Individually Identifiable Health Information. All health insurance plans, health care providers, and organizations that process medical information are bound by this law. Any information entered into the medical record is protected as well as any conversations that occur between health care providers. There must be strict policies in place to safe guard this information and limits are also put in place to restrict access to medical records. For example, in a hospital, many employees have access to computerized records. However, only the employees who are directly responsible for the patient's care are authorized to look at this information. Written permission is required for any information to be shared. Any violation of this law can be met with civil or criminal consequences.

99. B: When using a dishwasher, prewash is required to remove food particles from plates, silverware, and other items. The proper temperature for prewash is 110-140°F. The proper wash temperature is 140-160°F, and the proper rinse temperature is 170°F to ensure all dishes are properly sanitized. Correct placement of table wares is essential to proper cleaning in the dish machine. Some machines are equipped with hot air bow dry feature but many food service operations use air drying. This saves considerable energy. It is also important to have a service plan in place for the dish machine. This should include regular maintenance to ensure proper operation.

100. D: Universal precautions are methods to manage infection control by assuming all bodily fluids are infectious and could potentially contain HIV, HBV, or other dangerous infections. Bodily fluids include blood, secretions, saliva, etc. The use of gloves, masks, and/or gowns should be used if any contact with bodily fluids is expected. Frequent hand washing is also essential to controlling infections. The frequent use of alcohol-based hand sanitizer is also recommended, especially when moving between patients and from room to room.

101. C: Fire safety training is extremely important in food service establishments as there is a high risk of fire as well as potential for injury to employees, patients, and customers. Each food service establishment should have a fire safety policy that is reviewed with each employee at hiring and annually thereafter. The policy should include an evacuation route or plan. All employees should participate in mandatory fire drills to ensure they are prepared. Common causes of fires and types of fire extinguishers should be reviewed. Water-type extinguishers should never be used on a grease fire as this will cause the grease to splatter and increase the size of the fire very quickly. A very small grease fire can be put out by covering the pan with a lid. A class B fire extinguisher is appropriate for flammable liquids, such as grease, gasoline, or paints.

102. B: The Fair Labor Standards Act of 1938 was established to help prevent poverty. This law established minimum wage and was expanded in 1966 to include food service employees. The Equal Pay Act was an amendment to the Fair Labor Standards Act written in 1963. This law makes it illegal to discriminate on the basis of gender. Men and women must be paid the same wage for the same jobs if the jobs require similar skills and responsibilities. A wage difference can occur if it is based on seniority, merit, or other reasons besides gender.

103. A: Unemployment compensation is a national system that provides certain individuals with income during transitional times. It was established under the Social Security Act of 1935, and is a joint program between the federal government and the states. Many of the rules for unemployment compensation are subject to individual state guidelines. In general, unemployment compensation may be denied if an employee quit of his own volition and without provocation, or was dismissed due to unauthorized absences or misconduct. Eligibility requirements for unemployment compensation vary by state.

104. D: The food service director position for a large, tertiary care hospital is a very specialized position requiring advanced skill, experience, and knowledge. Thus, advertising the position in a small, weekly community newspaper is not likely to result in a pool of qualified applicants. Internal promotion of a current manager, who is familiar with the facility policy and operations, may be possible. That being said, it is wise to advertise the position using resources that reach large audiences, such as internet-based classifieds (Monster.com and others), newspapers, job placement recruiters, trade shows and job fairs, among others.

105. C: Employee retention can be bolstered by a variety of means. Great benefits packages and competitive compensations, with performance-based raises, are great motivational tools. Employee educational programs promote learning, future career growth, and possible promotions from within. Employees also like flexible work schedules. When this is not possible, manager consideration and accommodation of schedule requests go a long way towards satisfying employees. Moreover, the workplace should be characterized as a positive atmosphere to which employees can look forward to going each day.

106. C: The capital budget includes money for purchasing or replacing equipment and should be part of the long-term financial planning for an organization. Items included in the capital budget generally have a minimum dollar amount, such as $10 000. The operating budget serves the day-to-day operations. The cash budget accounts for incoming and outgoing cash. The master budget includes the capital, operating and cash budgets.

107. A: If labor costs are over budget, the manager needs to determine the cause of overspending by reviewing schedules, work flow, and production standards. Periods of down time should be avoided by assigning additional tasks for completion. The manager should also ensure that each employee is properly trained and performing at acceptable standards. The addition of self-serve stations, such as beverage centers or prepackaged sandwiches, may reduce workforce requirements. Another way to minimize labor costs is to review customer usage of services during open hours. If the service is not being utilized, it may be prudent to shorten the availability or discontinue the service.

108. D: Abraham Maslow developed a motivational theory based on individuals meeting certain growth needs before being able to advance to the next level. The first level is physiological need. This is the need to satisfy hunger, thirst, clothing, shelter, and breathing. Next, are safety needs, such as freedom from fear and harm. This is followed by social needs, such as the need to belong, be loved, have friends, and overall acceptance. The fourth need is satisfying self-esteem needs, such as status, recognition, or achievement. The last need is self-actualization where one reaches his or her own potential and is fulfilled. Maslow believed that the higher one got in the hierarchy, the more knowledge and wisdom one gained.

109. B: Kurt Lewin identified three styles of leadership in 1939. An autocratic leader is one who makes all the decisions without input from employees. This type of leadership style tends to produce the most dissatisfied employees. A decision made without the input of employees may set the employees up to fail if the decision is not a sound one. In a democratic style of leadership, the manager involves the employees in the decisions but reserves the right to make the final decision after reviewing input. This is usually a successful type of leadership unless opinions vary widely on all decisions. A laissez-faire style of leadership is one where the manager allows the employees to make the decisions but also makes the employees responsible for the consequences of that decision. This type of leadership style can work well with extremely motivated and knowledgeable employees.

110. D: In order to be an effective leader, good communication skills are essential. Communication can take various forms including oral, written, and action. The grapevine is indeed a form of communication; however, it is an informal method. Some facts may come through the grapevine, but most of the information has been skewed or altered. The grapevine also contains rumors or gossip and may be detrimental if the information is passed along. With effective communication, one is much more likely to remember what is being communicated. It is less likely an employee will remember something that is only verbalized and lacks visual or hands-on supplementation. Reading and understanding body language is also an important facet of good communication.

111. A: Merchandising is also known as marketing, promotions, and selling. Merchandising refers to product placement to help increase sales. In general, merchandising is all about making the product look better. For example, to merchandise a piece of fresh fruit, one might clean and polish the fruit, ensuring it has no bruises, then place the fruit in an attractive basket for eye-catching placement. Alternatively, fruits may be pre-plated with attractive garnishes. Likewise, weekly promotions, such as incorporating the item into various recipes, offering specialty items, and creatively using the item, may be an effective way of feature that item.

112. B: Branding is a marketing method that utilizes certain brands to increase sales. The brands can be nationally known or local brands. Retail item branding is a form of branding where the name of the product is strategically placed on the menu such that the menu reads Kellogg's Corn Flakes instead of just corn flakes. Restaurant branding is where nationally known restaurant chains are operating within a food service operation, such as in a hospital cafeteria or a school food service. In-house signature branding are special items created by the food service operation. These may be high quality sandwiches, salads, or other products. An entire marketing scheme, including logo and slogan development is then focused on the branding. Branding helps increase sales and revenue, and adds interest for the consumer.

113. C: The Joint Commission on the Accreditation of Healthcare Organizations has developed a list of abbreviations that should not be used in the medical record. This list is called the "Do Not Use" list. This list was developed in the interest of patient safety because frequent medical errors have been made using the abbreviations on this list. Some of the abbreviations on this list include: U (units) because it can be confused with a zero; and IU (international units) because it can be mistaken for intravenous. Trailing zeros should be omitted because the decimal point may be missing or illegible. QD and QOD should be written out as daily and every other day, respectively. MS needs to be written out because it can be interpreted to mean morphine sulfate or magnesium sulfate. Additional abbreviations may eventually be added to this list.

114. D: The National Restaurant Association sponsors the ServSafe program. This is a certification program that involves a training course and successful completion. The course may be offered online or at training sites. The certification is valid for 5 years. Concepts that are covered in this certification include dangers of food borne illness and how to prevent it. It also includes a review of personal hygiene. Other concepts include a review of food preparation, cross contamination, storage, serving, and pest management. The program helps managers stay updated with changes to the FDA Food Code. The training provides examples of situations to help participants apply the skills they are learning.

115. B: Employees can inadvertently be a cause of food borne illness. As a manager, there are a few situations to be aware of in terms of preventing potential food borne illness. These include employees who are touching the scalp or hair; wiping the nose or mouth; or coughing and sneezing into the hand. Other situations to be aware of include touching the skin where there may be a blemish or open wound that could be potentially infected, touching inside the ear, or spitting in the area where food is handled. Dirty uniforms are also a danger. Employee illness is sometimes difficult to gauge, but if fever is present at any time, the employee should be considered contagious and avoid coming to work. Proper hand washing, keeping oneself appropriately cleaned and groomed, and dressing in clean clothes are all training concerns.

116. D: A health inspector's visit should never be a complete surprise. Rather, it should be something that is planned and anticipated even if it is not scheduled. The food service operation should do self-assessments and self-inspections. The food service staff should be briefed on any findings so they can be addressed prior to an actual visit. When the health inspector visits, it is appropriate to ask to verify the inspector's credentials as there have been incidents of imposters. The inspection should never be refused because the inspector can then obtain a warrant to inspect the operation. Moreover, the initial refusal may raise a red flag to the inspector. It is appropriate to take notes during the inspection. Upon completion of the inspection, the report should be signed. Signing the report signifies only that you have received a copy; it does not mean you're going to be held responsible for what's on it.

117. B: The Food and Drug Administration (FDA) is responsible for publishing the Food Code. This code is updated every 4 years, but interim reports are published if new information needs to be addressed. The Food Code is scientifically-based and applies to all public establishments where food is involved, including restaurants, grocery stores, and institutional food services. It provides useful and realistic information on preventing food borne illness. Topics addressed by the Food Code are food, equipment, utensils, lines, physical facilities, and plumbing and water issues. It also addresses personnel in terms of cleanliness, proper hygiene, and the use of clean clothing. It does not directly establish specify uniforms or clothing criteria. The Food Code also addresses supervisory issues to help prevent illness from spreading. It is a comprehensive report full of important information.

118. A: The JCAHO has started using tracer methodology to track a patient throughout their entire hospital experience. A patient is identified and the course of care is followed. The tracer may include observation of patient care, medication dispensing, and care planning. The patient of the family may be interviewed. Medical records are reviewed and old records may be requested. The interaction, training, and development of the staff are reviewed. Policies and procedures may be reviewed. The tracer may involve review of the entire patient stay, to include interdepartmental evaluations. Nutrition care and food service is an integral part of the survey as well.

119. C: The National Patient Safety Goals were developed by JCAHO in an effort to improve patient safety. It also incorporates Universal Protocol, which involves a 3-step process to ensure the correct body part is treated. There are 16 patient safety goals that include improved communication, such as how verbal orders are treated and the use of the "Do Not Use" list. The goals also involve using two patient identifiers, such as the ID band and asking the patient for their name. Furthermore, the goals target medication labeling, nomenclature, and reconciliation. The goals also encourage the patient to be actively involved in their own care by asking questions or having family members involved as a safety check.

120. B: The process of benchmarking is an aspect of quality improvement initiatives. Benchmarking is the process where the performance of one group is measured against a comparable group. Sometimes performance is measured against national standards. The most useful type of benchmarking is comparing oneself against the best possible group, who have set and maintained high goals and standards. The process by which they have achieved the standards is closely examined. The process helps organizations identify their strengths and weaknesses. The Leapfrog Group and Press Ganey are two groups that collect this type of data. The Leapfrog Group looks at patient safety issues, whereas Press Ganey looks at patient satisfaction, safety, the flow of patients, food service, and other areas. Food service operations can use this information to improve their operations.

121. C: In order for the quality improvement process to work, there must be measurable outcomes. Outcomes are the end result of interventions. Outcomes can encompass clinical, functional, or financial issues. The outcome needs to be objective and measurable. Perception also plays a role in outcomes. In the examples above, measuring and tracking the percentage of patients who met 100% of their nutrient needs may be a difficult outcome to measure, especially in a large facility. This would be time consuming and labor intensive. It would also include some degree of uncertainty, due to the estimations that would be made.

122. D: The Institute of Medicine (IOM) published a report in 2001, called Crossing the Quality Chasm: A New Health System for the 21st Century. In this report, the IOM stated that the US healthcare system needed to undergo significant changes in order to improve the quality of healthcare. It identified 6 aims for improving healthcare. These include patient safety, patient centered, effectiveness, efficiency, timeliness, and equity. An example of patient safety might be avoiding central line placement unless parenteral nutrition is required for more than a week. An example of patient centeredness is ensuring patients who go home on home enteral feeding receive a feeding schedule that works for their situation. An example of effectiveness might be using protocols to address hyperglycemia in hospitalized patients. An example of efficiency might include automatically advancing tube feedings based on tolerance. Timeliness might include completing all nutrition screens within 24 hours.

123. A: The ADA's Standards of Professional Performance (SOPP) were written for RDs and DTRs who work in a variety of settings. The standards reflect the behavior expected of a professional. There is a minimum competency level that must be achieved. There are 6 areas of professional behavior that are applicable, and these areas include: service provision, applying research, applying knowledge and using communication, allocating resources, quality, and competence. SOPP also addresses the supervision of DTRs by RDs. The RD is ultimately accountable for care provided by the DTR. The RD is in charge of the nutrition care process (NCP) but can delegate appropriate tasks to the DTR.

124. D: The DTR who is involved with the nutritional care of patients must work under the supervision of an RD. If this is not being done, state agencies may investigate, and it could lead to the loss of an RD's license, fines for the facility, loss of the facility's license, or certification status for reimbursement. For end stage renal disease, the Centers for Medicare and Medicaid Services state that all nutritional care must be provided by an RD who has at least one year of experience post-internship. Much of healthcare is controlled at the state level, thus definitions of certain terms must be verified in the appropriate state. The scope of a DTR's practice varies by state, but may include screening, collecting data, diet histories, or calorie counts.

125. C: There are many job opportunities for DTRs. Some jobs require the DTR to work as part of a team under the supervision of the RD. These jobs are often found in settings such as hospitals, nursing homes, long-term care facilities, and research environments. Other jobs enable the DTR to work independently but still with the supervision of an RD. The jobs may be found in business, health clubs, or contract food service companies. DTRs can educate people, such as new moms in the WIC program or clients in a health club, who need help with weight loss. DTRs also work in schools, correctional facilities, and other settings. Moreover, DTRs may also work in a management capacity supervising employees, developing budgets, purchasing, etc.

126. B: The Code of Ethics was implemented to provide direction to dietetic professionals for issues surrounding practice and conduct. The code applies to any member of the American Dietetic Association (ADA). Even RDs and DTRs who are not ADA members, must comply with the code, except for the points relating to membership. The Code of Ethics is built on the foundation that all dietetic professionals should always be honest, fair, and display integrity. The code states that a practitioner should not practice if he is struggling with an active addiction, is mentally incompetent, or has impaired judgment. The code addresses the relationship with clients, to the overall profession, and to other dietetic professionals. A committee reviews reported ethical violations. In the above example, an RD who is accepting money from a physician group to promote the use of their products is likely committing an ethical violation.

127. C: A DTR has the responsibility to help clients decipher available nutrition information. Many factors must be considered when interpreting literature, whether it is publicized via a peer-reviewed journal or a media outlet. Media will often sensationalize a story. Literature may present information that is not statistically significant or has study design flaws. Moreover, studies may not have examined endpoints, such as the development of a disease. Instead, they may measure certain markers that do not always translate into the development of a disease. It is also important to note that some studies are done on animals, and the data may not be relevant to human nutrition.

128. A: Randomized controlled trials (RCT) are considered to be the gold standard in evidenced-based practice. The design of these studies requires subjects to be randomly assigned to groups. When subjects are divided into groups and neither the subject nor the researcher know what group the individuals are in, the study is double-blind. Double-blind studies are particularly reliable as they eliminate researcher and/or participant bias.

Cohort studies examine data collected from a large group over a period of time. Good data can be obtained from these types of studies.

Case controlled studies compare one group of people who already have certain symptoms or a specific disease to a similar group without the same trait. These studies cannot analyze past data, such as diet, because the information has not been collected. A consensus statement is a statement made public by a group after reviewing research.

129. B: A performance appraisal is an evaluation of an employee's job performance. A yearly performance appraisal is required by the Joint Commission on the Accreditation of Healthcare Organizations (JCAHO) for DTRs. Performance appraisals are not only an evaluation but also an opportunity for the employee to discuss job expectations, review strengths and weakness, and examine areas for improvement. It is also a way to indicate the desire for growth within the organization and to develop a plan to achieve this. Training issues should also be reviewed. Any negative feedback discussed in the performance appraisal should not be news to the employee as performance issues should be addressed as soon as they become concerning. Performance appraisals may coincide with salary adjustments.

How to Overcome Test Anxiety

Just the thought of taking a test is enough to make most people a little nervous. A test is an important event that can have a long-term impact on your future, so it's important to take it seriously and it's natural to feel anxious about performing well. But just because anxiety is normal, that doesn't mean that it's helpful in test taking, or that you should simply accept it as part of your life. Anxiety can have a variety of effects. These effects can be mild, like making you feel slightly nervous, or severe, like blocking your ability to focus or remember even a simple detail.

If you experience test anxiety—whether severe or mild—it's important to know how to beat it. To discover this, first you need to understand what causes test anxiety.

Causes of Test Anxiety

While we often think of anxiety as an uncontrollable emotional state, it can actually be caused by simple, practical things. One of the most common causes of test anxiety is that a person does not feel adequately prepared for their test. This feeling can be the result of many different issues such as poor study habits or lack of organization, but the most common culprit is time management. Starting to study too late, failing to organize your study time to cover all of the material, or being distracted while you study will mean that you're not well prepared for the test. This may lead to cramming the night before, which will cause you to be physically and mentally exhausted for the test. Poor time management also contributes to feelings of stress, fear, and hopelessness as you realize you are not well prepared but don't know what to do about it.

Other times, test anxiety is not related to your preparation for the test but comes from unresolved fear. This may be a past failure on a test, or poor performance on tests in general. It may come from comparing yourself to others who seem to be performing better or from the stress of living up to expectations. Anxiety may be driven by fears of the future—how failure on this test would affect your educational and career goals. These fears are often completely irrational, but they can still negatively impact your test performance.

> **Review Video: 3 Reasons You Have Test Anxiety**
> Visit mometrix.com/academy and enter code: 428468

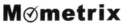

Elements of Test Anxiety

As mentioned earlier, test anxiety is considered to be an emotional state, but it has physical and mental components as well. Sometimes you may not even realize that you are suffering from test anxiety until you notice the physical symptoms. These can include trembling hands, rapid heartbeat, sweating, nausea, and tense muscles. Extreme anxiety may lead to fainting or vomiting. Obviously, any of these symptoms can have a negative impact on testing. It is important to recognize them as soon as they begin to occur so that you can address the problem before it damages your performance.

> **Review Video: 3 Ways to Tell You Have Test Anxiety**
> Visit mometrix.com/academy and enter code: 927847

The mental components of test anxiety include trouble focusing and inability to remember learned information. During a test, your mind is on high alert, which can help you recall information and stay focused for an extended period of time. However, anxiety interferes with your mind's natural processes, causing you to blank out, even on the questions you know well. The strain of testing during anxiety makes it difficult to stay focused, especially on a test that may take several hours. Extreme anxiety can take a huge mental toll, making it difficult not only to recall test information but even to understand the test questions or pull your thoughts together.

> **Review Video: How Test Anxiety Affects Memory**
> Visit mometrix.com/academy and enter code: 609003

Effects of Test Anxiety

Test anxiety is like a disease—if left untreated, it will get progressively worse. Anxiety leads to poor performance, and this reinforces the feelings of fear and failure, which in turn lead to poor performances on subsequent tests. It can grow from a mild nervousness to a crippling condition. If allowed to progress, test anxiety can have a big impact on your schooling, and consequently on your future.

Test anxiety can spread to other parts of your life. Anxiety on tests can become anxiety in any stressful situation, and blanking on a test can turn into panicking in a job situation. But fortunately, you don't have to let anxiety rule your testing and determine your grades. There are a number of relatively simple steps you can take to move past anxiety and function normally on a test and in the rest of life.

> **Review Video: How Test Anxiety Impacts Your Grades**
> Visit mometrix.com/academy and enter code: 939819

Physical Steps for Beating Test Anxiety

While test anxiety is a serious problem, the good news is that it can be overcome. It doesn't have to control your ability to think and remember information. While it may take time, you can begin taking steps today to beat anxiety.

Just as your first hint that you may be struggling with anxiety comes from the physical symptoms, the first step to treating it is also physical. Rest is crucial for having a clear, strong mind. If you are tired, it is much easier to give in to anxiety. But if you establish good sleep habits, your body and mind will be ready to perform optimally, without the strain of exhaustion. Additionally, sleeping well helps you to retain information better, so you're more likely to recall the answers when you see the test questions.

Getting good sleep means more than going to bed on time. It's important to allow your brain time to relax. Take study breaks from time to time so it doesn't get overworked, and don't study right before bed. Take time to rest your mind before trying to rest your body, or you may find it difficult to fall asleep.

> **Review Video: The Importance of Sleep for Your Brain**
> Visit mometrix.com/academy and enter code: 319338

Along with sleep, other aspects of physical health are important in preparing for a test. Good nutrition is vital for good brain function. Sugary foods and drinks may give a burst of energy but this burst is followed by a crash, both physically and emotionally. Instead, fuel your body with protein and vitamin-rich foods.

Also, drink plenty of water. Dehydration can lead to headaches and exhaustion, especially if your brain is already under stress from the rigors of the test. Particularly if your test is a long one, drink water during the breaks. And if possible, take an energy-boosting snack to eat between sections.

> **Review Video: How Diet Can Affect your Mood**
> Visit mometrix.com/academy and enter code: 624317

Along with sleep and diet, a third important part of physical health is exercise. Maintaining a steady workout schedule is helpful, but even taking 5-minute study breaks to walk can help get your blood pumping faster and clear your head. Exercise also releases endorphins, which contribute to a positive feeling and can help combat test anxiety.

When you nurture your physical health, you are also contributing to your mental health. If your body is healthy, your mind is much more likely to be healthy as well. So take time to rest, nourish your body with healthy food and water, and get moving as much as possible. Taking these physical steps will make you stronger and more able to take the mental steps necessary to overcome test anxiety.

> **Review Video: How to Stay Healthy and Prevent Test Anxiety**
> Visit mometrix.com/academy and enter code: 877894

Mental Steps for Beating Test Anxiety

Working on the mental side of test anxiety can be more challenging, but as with the physical side, there are clear steps you can take to overcome it. As mentioned earlier, test anxiety often stems from lack of preparation, so the obvious solution is to prepare for the test. Effective studying may be the most important weapon you have for beating test anxiety, but you can and should employ several other mental tools to combat fear.

First, boost your confidence by reminding yourself of past success—tests or projects that you aced. If you're putting as much effort into preparing for this test as you did for those, there's no reason you should expect to fail here. Work hard to prepare; then trust your preparation.

Second, surround yourself with encouraging people. It can be helpful to find a study group, but be sure that the people you're around will encourage a positive attitude. If you spend time with others who are anxious or cynical, this will only contribute to your own anxiety. Look for others who are motivated to study hard from a desire to succeed, not from a fear of failure.

Third, reward yourself. A test is physically and mentally tiring, even without anxiety, and it can be helpful to have something to look forward to. Plan an activity following the test, regardless of the outcome, such as going to a movie or getting ice cream.

When you are taking the test, if you find yourself beginning to feel anxious, remind yourself that you know the material. Visualize successfully completing the test. Then take a few deep, relaxing breaths and return to it. Work through the questions carefully but with confidence, knowing that you are capable of succeeding.

Developing a healthy mental approach to test taking will also aid in other areas of life. Test anxiety affects more than just the actual test—it can be damaging to your mental health and even contribute to depression. It's important to beat test anxiety before it becomes a problem for more than testing.

> **Review Video: Test Anxiety and Depression**
> Visit mometrix.com/academy and enter code: 904704

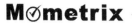

Study Strategy

Being prepared for the test is necessary to combat anxiety, but what does being prepared look like? You may study for hours on end and still not feel prepared. What you need is a strategy for test prep. The next few pages outline our recommended steps to help you plan out and conquer the challenge of preparation.

STEP 1: SCOPE OUT THE TEST

Learn everything you can about the format (multiple choice, essay, etc.) and what will be on the test. Gather any study materials, course outlines, or sample exams that may be available. Not only will this help you to prepare, but knowing what to expect can help to alleviate test anxiety.

STEP 2: MAP OUT THE MATERIAL

Look through the textbook or study guide and make note of how many chapters or sections it has. Then divide these over the time you have. For example, if a book has 15 chapters and you have five days to study, you need to cover three chapters each day. Even better, if you have the time, leave an extra day at the end for overall review after you have gone through the material in depth.

If time is limited, you may need to prioritize the material. Look through it and make note of which sections you think you already have a good grasp on, and which need review. While you are studying, skim quickly through the familiar sections and take more time on the challenging parts. Write out your plan so you don't get lost as you go. Having a written plan also helps you feel more in control of the study, so anxiety is less likely to arise from feeling overwhelmed at the amount to cover.

STEP 3: GATHER YOUR TOOLS

Decide what study method works best for you. Do you prefer to highlight in the book as you study and then go back over the highlighted portions? Or do you type out notes of the important information? Or is it helpful to make flashcards that you can carry with you? Assemble the pens, index cards, highlighters, post-it notes, and any other materials you may need so you won't be distracted by getting up to find things while you study.

If you're having a hard time retaining the information or organizing your notes, experiment with different methods. For example, try color-coding by subject with colored pens, highlighters, or post-it notes. If you learn better by hearing, try recording yourself reading your notes so you can listen while in the car, working out, or simply sitting at your desk. Ask a friend to quiz you from your flashcards, or try teaching someone the material to solidify it in your mind.

STEP 4: CREATE YOUR ENVIRONMENT

It's important to avoid distractions while you study. This includes both the obvious distractions like visitors and the subtle distractions like an uncomfortable chair (or a too-comfortable couch that makes you want to fall asleep). Set up the best study environment possible: good lighting and a comfortable work area. If background music helps you focus, you may want to turn it on, but otherwise keep the room quiet. If you are using a computer to take notes, be sure you don't have any other windows open, especially applications like social media, games, or anything else that could distract you. Silence your phone and turn off notifications. Be sure to keep water close by so you stay hydrated while you study (but avoid unhealthy drinks and snacks).

Also, take into account the best time of day to study. Are you freshest first thing in the morning? Try to set aside some time then to work through the material. Is your mind clearer in the afternoon or evening? Schedule your study session then. Another method is to study at the same time of day that you will take the test, so that your brain gets used to working on the material at that time and will be ready to focus at test time.

STEP 5: STUDY!

Once you have done all the study preparation, it's time to settle into the actual studying. Sit down, take a few moments to settle your mind so you can focus, and begin to follow your study plan. Don't give in to distractions or let yourself procrastinate. This is your time to prepare so you'll be ready to fearlessly approach the test. Make the most of the time and stay focused.

Of course, you don't want to burn out. If you study too long you may find that you're not retaining the information very well. Take regular study breaks. For example, taking five minutes out of every hour to walk briskly, breathing deeply and swinging your arms, can help your mind stay fresh.

As you get to the end of each chapter or section, it's a good idea to do a quick review. Remind yourself of what you learned and work on any difficult parts. When you feel that you've mastered the material, move on to the next part. At the end of your study session, briefly skim through your notes again.

But while review is helpful, cramming last minute is NOT. If at all possible, work ahead so that you won't need to fit all your study into the last day. Cramming overloads your brain with more information than it can process and retain, and your tired mind may struggle to recall even previously learned information when it is overwhelmed with last-minute study. Also, the urgent nature of cramming and the stress placed on your brain contribute to anxiety. You'll be more likely to go to the test feeling unprepared and having trouble thinking clearly.

So don't cram, and don't stay up late before the test, even just to review your notes at a leisurely pace. Your brain needs rest more than it needs to go over the information again. In fact, plan to finish your studies by noon or early afternoon the day before the test. Give your brain the rest of the day to relax or focus on other things, and get a good night's sleep. Then you will be fresh for the test and better able to recall what you've studied.

STEP 6: TAKE A PRACTICE TEST

Many courses offer sample tests, either online or in the study materials. This is an excellent resource to check whether you have mastered the material, as well as to prepare for the test format and environment.

Check the test format ahead of time: the number of questions, the type (multiple choice, free response, etc.), and the time limit. Then create a plan for working through them. For example, if you have 30 minutes to take a 60-question test, your limit is 30 seconds per question. Spend less time on the questions you know well so that you can take more time on the difficult ones.

If you have time to take several practice tests, take the first one open book, with no time limit. Work through the questions at your own pace and make sure you fully understand them. Gradually work up to taking a test under test conditions: sit at a desk with all study materials put away and set a timer. Pace yourself to make sure you finish the test with time to spare and go back to check your answers if you have time.

After each test, check your answers. On the questions you missed, be sure you understand why you missed them. Did you misread the question (tests can use tricky wording)? Did you forget the information? Or was it something you hadn't learned? Go back and study any shaky areas that the practice tests reveal.

Taking these tests not only helps with your grade, but also aids in combating test anxiety. If you're already used to the test conditions, you're less likely to worry about it, and working through tests until you're scoring well gives you a confidence boost. Go through the practice tests until you feel comfortable, and then you can go into the test knowing that you're ready for it.

Test Tips

On test day, you should be confident, knowing that you've prepared well and are ready to answer the questions. But aside from preparation, there are several test day strategies you can employ to maximize your performance.

First, as stated before, get a good night's sleep the night before the test (and for several nights before that, if possible). Go into the test with a fresh, alert mind rather than staying up late to study.

Try not to change too much about your normal routine on the day of the test. It's important to eat a nutritious breakfast, but if you normally don't eat breakfast at all, consider eating just a protein bar. If you're a coffee drinker, go ahead and have your normal coffee. Just make sure you time it so that the caffeine doesn't wear off right in the middle of your test. Avoid sugary beverages, and drink enough water to stay hydrated but not so much that you need a restroom break 10 minutes into the test. If your test isn't first thing in the morning, consider going for a walk or doing a light workout before the test to get your blood flowing.

Allow yourself enough time to get ready, and leave for the test with plenty of time to spare so you won't have the anxiety of scrambling to arrive in time. Another reason to be early is to select a good seat. It's helpful to sit away from doors and windows, which can be distracting. Find a good seat, get out your supplies, and settle your mind before the test begins.

When the test begins, start by going over the instructions carefully, even if you already know what to expect. Make sure you avoid any careless mistakes by following the directions.

Then begin working through the questions, pacing yourself as you've practiced. If you're not sure on an answer, don't spend too much time on it, and don't let it shake your confidence. Either skip it and come back later, or eliminate as many wrong answers as possible and guess among the remaining ones. Don't dwell on these questions as you continue—put them out of your mind and focus on what lies ahead.

Be sure to read all of the answer choices, even if you're sure the first one is the right answer. Sometimes you'll find a better one if you keep reading. But don't second-guess yourself if you do immediately know the answer. Your gut instinct is usually right. Don't let test anxiety rob you of the information you know.

If you have time at the end of the test (and if the test format allows), go back and review your answers. Be cautious about changing any, since your first instinct tends to be correct, but make sure you didn't misread any of the questions or accidentally mark the wrong answer choice. Look over any you skipped and make an educated guess.

At the end, leave the test feeling confident. You've done your best, so don't waste time worrying about your performance or wishing you could change anything. Instead, celebrate the successful completion of this test. And finally, use this test to learn how to deal with anxiety even better next time.

> **Review Video: 5 Tips to Beat Test Anxiety**
> Visit mometrix.com/academy and enter code: 570656

Important Qualification

Not all anxiety is created equal. If your test anxiety is causing major issues in your life beyond the classroom or testing center, or if you are experiencing troubling physical symptoms related to your anxiety, it may be a sign of a serious physiological or psychological condition. If this sounds like your situation, we strongly encourage you to seek professional help.

Thank You

We at Mometrix would like to extend our heartfelt thanks to you, our friend and patron, for allowing us to play a part in your journey. It is a privilege to serve people from all walks of life who are unified in their commitment to building the best future they can for themselves.

The preparation you devote to these important testing milestones may be the most valuable educational opportunity you have for making a real difference in your life. We encourage you to put your heart into it—that feeling of succeeding, overcoming, and yes, conquering will be well worth the hours you've invested.

We want to hear your story, your struggles and your successes, and if you see any opportunities for us to improve our materials so we can help others even more effectively in the future, please share that with us as well. **The team at Mometrix would be absolutely thrilled to hear from you!** So please, send us an email (support@mometrix.com) and let's stay in touch.

If you'd like some additional help, check out these other resources we offer for your exam:
http://MometrixFlashcards.com/RD

Additional Bonus Material

Due to our efforts to try to keep this book to a manageable length, we've created a link that will give you access to all of your additional bonus material.

Please visit https://www.mometrix.com/bonus948/dtr to access the information.